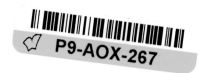
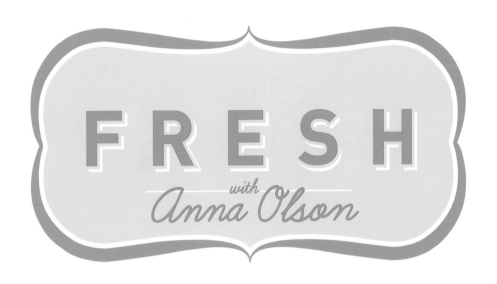

FRESH

with
Anna Olson

whitecap

Copyright © 2009 by Peace Point
    Entertainment Group and Anna Olson
Whitecap Books

Whitecap Books is known for its expertise in the cookbook market, and has produced some of the most innovative and familiar titles found in kitchens across North America. Visit our website at www.whitecap.ca.

Edited by Lesley Cameron
Proofread by Grace Yaginuma
Cover design by Michelle Mayne and
    Mauve Pagé
Interior design by Setareh Ashrafologhalai
Food photography by Ryan Szulc
    (www.ryanszulc.ca)
Food styling by Anna Olson
Assistant food styling by Lisa Rollo
Prop styling by Madeleine Johari

Printed in Canada

Library and Archives Canada Cataloguing in Publication

Olson, Anna, 1968–
    Fresh with Anna Olson.

ISBN 978-1-55285-995-7

    1. Cookery. I. Title.

TX714.O484 2009   641.5
C2009-902674-0

The publisher acknowledges the financial sup-port of the Government of Canada through the Book Publishing Industry Development Program (BPIDP) and the Province of British Columbia through the Book Publishing Tax Credit.

09 10 11 12 13   5 4 3 2 1

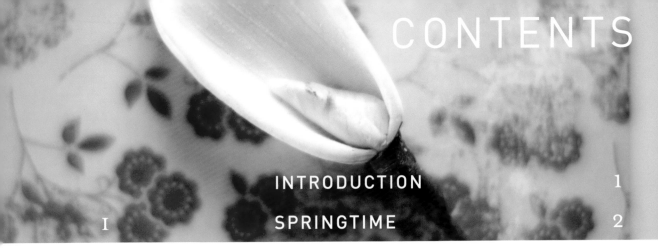

CONTENTS

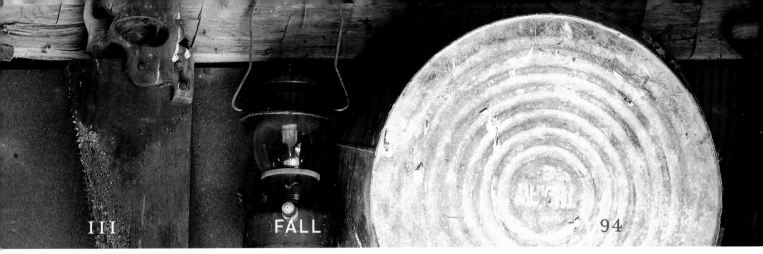

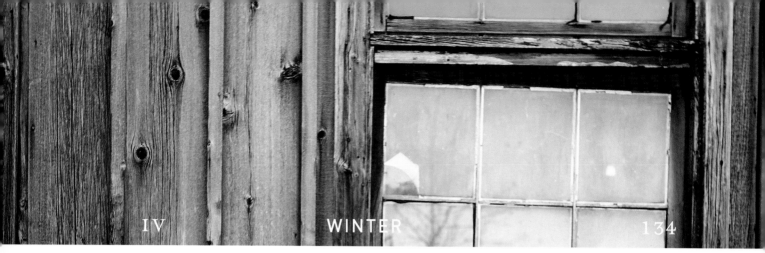

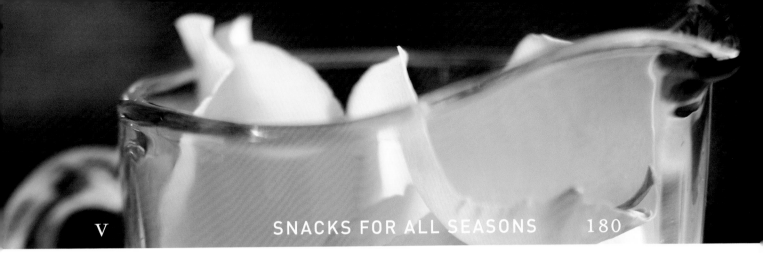

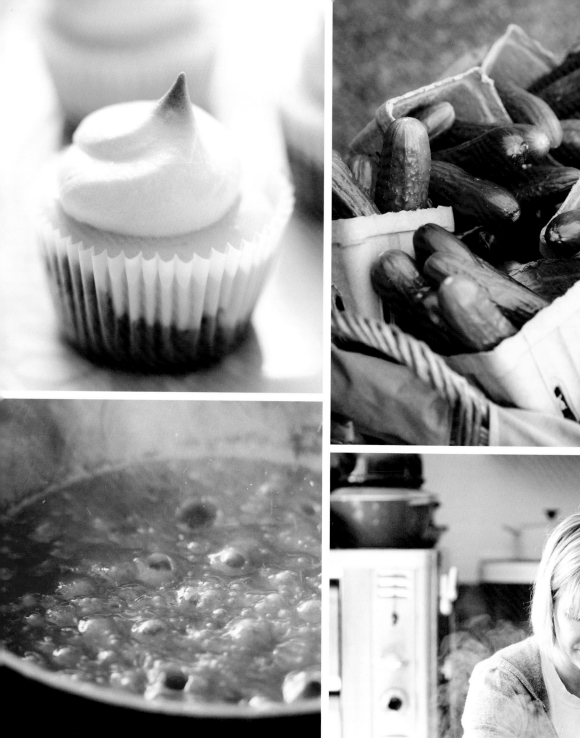
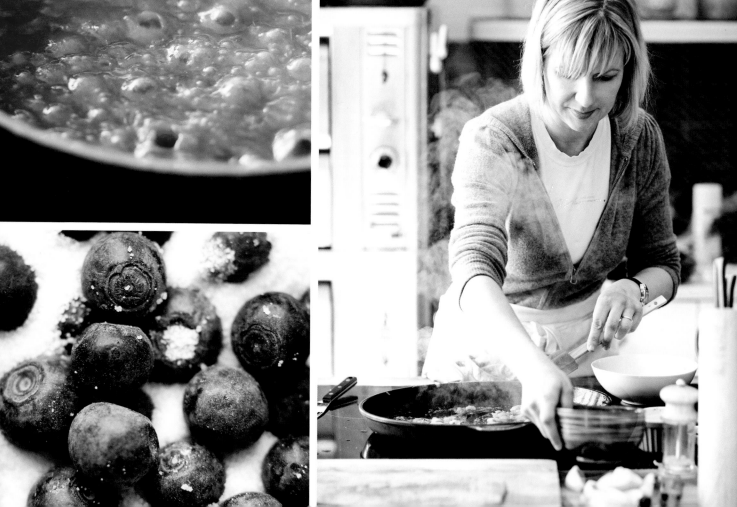

I am often asked, "What is your favorite dish to make?" And my answer is always the same: "It depends what time of year it is."

I am a seasonally motivated cook. It is the foods available at their peak, the cooking techniques of the season, and my own personal cravings that dictate what I make to satisfy myself and others. And the things I make shape my culinary identity.

Everyone who cooks has one. It is something that constantly changes and grows just as a person changes and grows. A long list of things influences the food we end up making, hence shaping our culinary identity. Some of the most basic influences are

- our cultural heritage
- the time and place in which we live
- our access to ingredients
- how much time we have
- our personal tastes and dietary needs

Like our personalities, or even DNA, a culinary identity is unique to each one of us. But we are undeniably linked to and bonded with one another, and food forges that bond. When we come together to eat with family and friends, we share not just conversation over the table but also an enjoyment of what we are eating. How many of our fond memories are tied to occasions where food is involved, and are of helping to put together a meal?

If you've watched my show of the same name, *Fresh with Anna Olson*, you know that I often share some of the "meal memories" I have enjoyed with family and friends. What has always made eating together even more special to me is the journey from idea to reality—the process of getting delicious creations to the table. I get so excited about planning a meal, finding the ingredients that I know my guests will like, and spending time in the kitchen cooking and creating.

A valuable aspect of creating these meals has been thinking about how to best capture the season. And it's always about cooking with fresh, local ingredients—which is not just a trend. It is the way we used to cook and eat in the days before our modern food industry made it common for food to be transported long distances. To cook with the seasons makes menu building simple, since food that *grows together, goes together* makes flavor pairings logical. And shopping for locally grown or locally produced ingredients means buying food at its best, meant to be eaten right away.

Wherever you may live, there are opportunities to source out local and seasonal ingredients. It's not just limited to shopping at farm-gate stands. Many towns and cities now offer farmers' markets, and the number of independent producers of cheeses, meats, preserves, and even ice cream continues to grow.

I hope you enjoy this cookbook. I will take it as a personal compliment if even just a few of these recipes work themselves into becoming part of your culinary identity.

SPRINGTIME

Springtime is about color. After a season of gray—gray skies, gray barren trees, gray sweaters, and gray pallor (unless we have a chance to escape to somewhere tropical for a week!)—the first signs of new growth can almost take us by surprise.

The first greens of spring are so bright—chives shooting up through decaying leaves, shoots of mint popping up where they weren't the year before. There's also a certain fragility to spring. Because it's so new, we have to treat its first few flavors delicately.

Fresh cheeses like goat cheese and ricotta figure prominently now as their mild character doesn't overwhelm the new produce. The season for caramelized onions has passed. It's time to enjoy vegetables from your own garden, or start making the Saturday morning trip to the farmers' market part of your weekly shopping routine. Always remember: what grows together, goes together. Spring herbs like chives, mint, and tarragon magically intertwine with snow peas, garden peas, and spinach.

Open your kitchen window, take a deep breath, and let your appetite guide you.

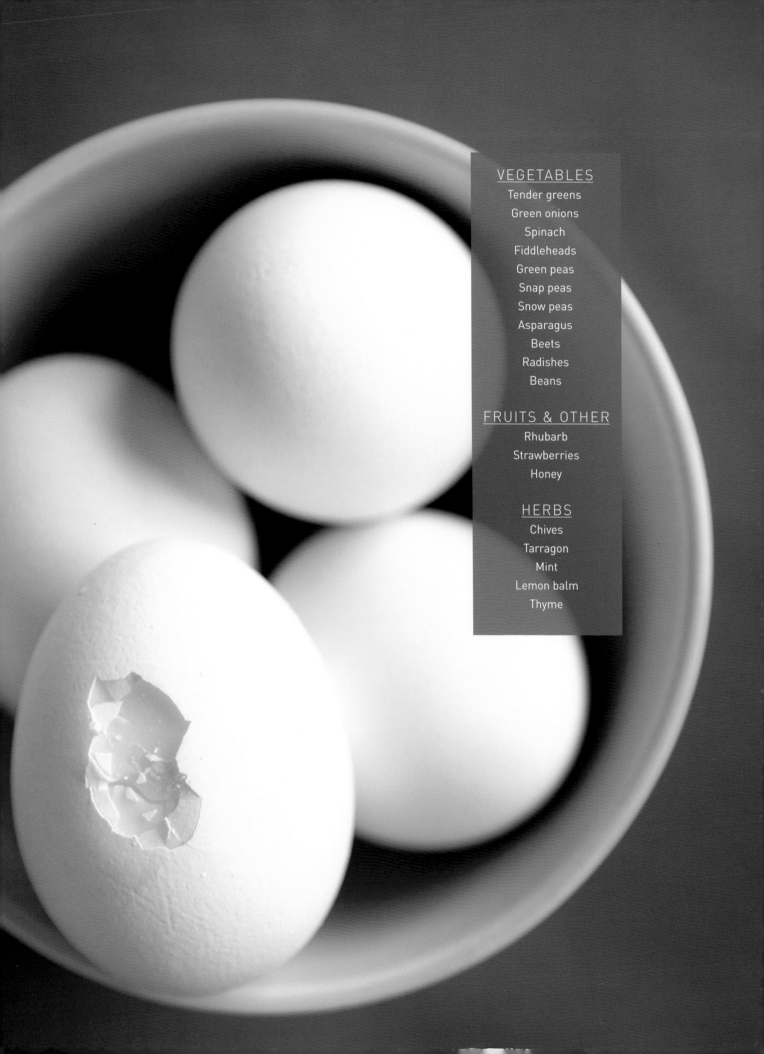

VEGETABLES
Tender greens
Green onions
Spinach
Fiddleheads
Green peas
Snap peas
Snow peas
Asparagus
Beets
Radishes
Beans

FRUITS & OTHER
Rhubarb
Strawberries
Honey

HERBS
Chives
Tarragon
Mint
Lemon balm
Thyme

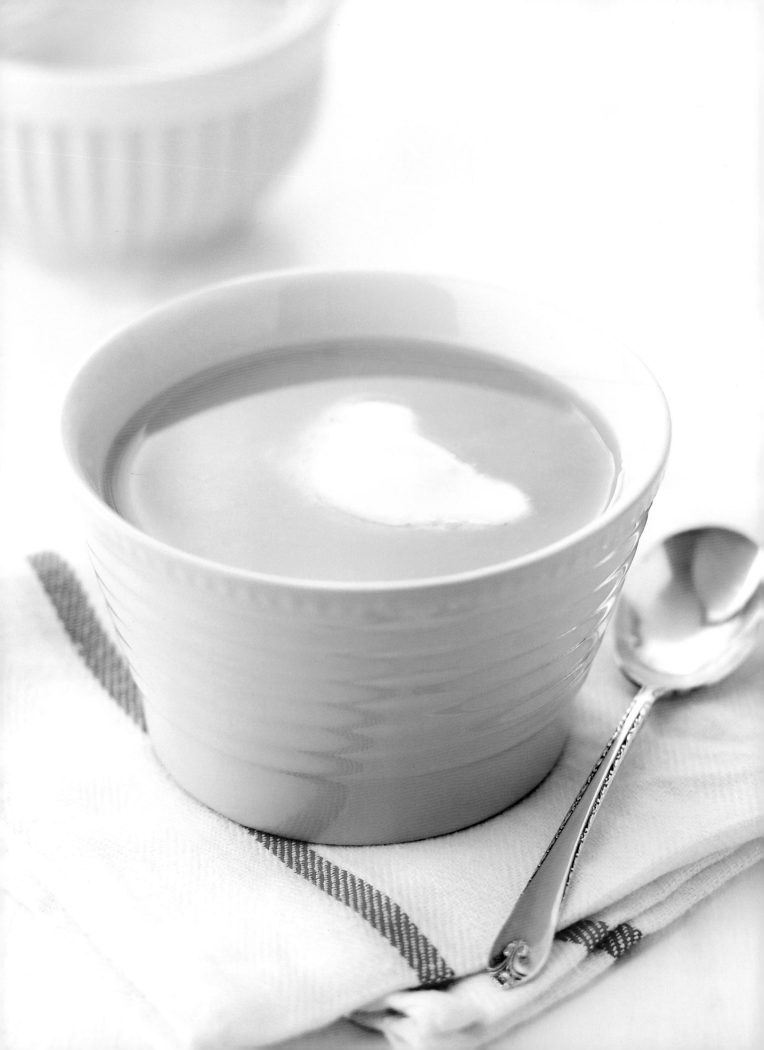

SPRING PEA SOUP with MINT *Serves 10 to 12*

This soup embraces spring when prepared with fresh peas, but it's equally satisfying in winter, made with frozen peas.

FRESH TAKE

- Warm or chilled, this soup is tasty. The key is to taste it at the temperature at which it is to be served. Chilling the soup mutes some of the flavors, including salt, so taste it once it's chilled (after having seasoned and tasted it warm) to see if the seasoning needs adjusting.

- Served hot, this soup holds its bright green color for only about 20 minutes, so serve it right away. To chill the soup and keep it green, pour it (or strain it) into a bowl nested in a larger bowl filled with ice. Stir the soup gently until cool then chill it immediately.

- Even though the soup is a vibrant green color, I call for only the white and light green parts of the leeks. The flavor of the darker green part of the leeks is tasty in stock or under a roasting chicken, but it never becomes quite tender enough to eat, even when cooked slowly.

1 Tbsp	butter or olive oil	15 mL
1½ cups	chopped leeks, white and light green parts only	375 mL
2 cups	peeled and diced Yukon Gold potatoes	500 mL
8 cups	chicken or vegetable stock	2 L
splash	dry vermouth	splash
3 cups	fresh or frozen green peas	750 mL
2 sprigs each	fresh thyme, mint, and tarragon	2 sprigs each
	salt & pepper	
	sour cream or crème fraîche, for garnish	

In a large pot, heat the butter or olive oil over medium heat. Add the leeks and sweat them until soft, about 6 minutes, stirring often. Add the potato, stock, and vermouth, and bring up to a simmer. Cook until the potatoes are tender, about 15 minutes. Add the peas and sprigs of herb (tying them with a string to keep them together). Bring this just up to a simmer. Remove the herbs and purée the soup until smooth. Strain through a sieve for a smoother soup (optional) then season to taste and serve immediately garnished with sour cream or crème fraîche.

This soup is also lovely served chilled and topped with baby shrimp, crab, or chopped avocado.

FIDDLEHEAD SALAD with PICKLED RED ONIONS & MAPLE TOASTED PECANS *Serves 6*

A magical combination of varied colors and textures builds a salad that reaches new heights of complexity without being complicated. The three main elements that create such harmony are all delectable and versatile on their own.

FRESH TAKE

- A fiddlehead embodies all that is spring. Small and delicate, these curly fern shoots are mild and have an almost creamy taste similar to artichoke hearts. It's worth noting that fiddleheads should only be eaten once cooked—blanching removes something called *shikimic acid* (long story short, an acid that is transformed and used in flu medications, but not meant to be consumed in its raw form).

- If you can't find fiddleheads, don't panic. You can use freshly cooked artichoke hearts or even blanched snap peas instead.

- Fiddleheads grow in damp forest beds and they take a bit of the forest with them when picked. If using fresh, take the time to soak and gently clean them. Frozen fiddleheads are already cleaned.

- The pickled red onions make a great condiment for burgers, grilled fish, or chicken, while the maple toasted pecans are a nice diversion on a cheese plate or even sprinkled on an apple tart or ice cream. Talk about versatile!

PICKLED RED ONIONS
Makes about 4 cups (1 ℓ)

4 cups	sliced red onions	1 L
⅓ cup	sugar	80 mL
⅓ cup	honey	80 mL
1 cup	dry white wine	250 mL
¼ cup	lemon juice	60 mL
1 tsp	salt	5 mL

Simmer all the ingredients, uncovered, over medium heat until the onions are tender and the liquid has evaporated, about 10 minutes. These can be refrigerated for up to 6 weeks.

MAPLE TOASTED PECANS
Makes 2 cups (500 ml)

2 cups	pecan halves	500 mL
3 Tbsp	pure maple syrup	45 mL
1 tsp	ground black pepper	5 mL

Preheat the oven to 350°F (180°C). Line a baking tray with parchment paper.

Toss the pecans with the maple syrup and black pepper to coat. Spread the pecans on the prepared tray and bake them for 10 to 12 minutes, without stirring, until toasted. Let cool in the pan. As the maple syrup cools it will caramelize onto the pecans.

The pecans can be stored in an airtight container for up to 1 month.

Continued . . .

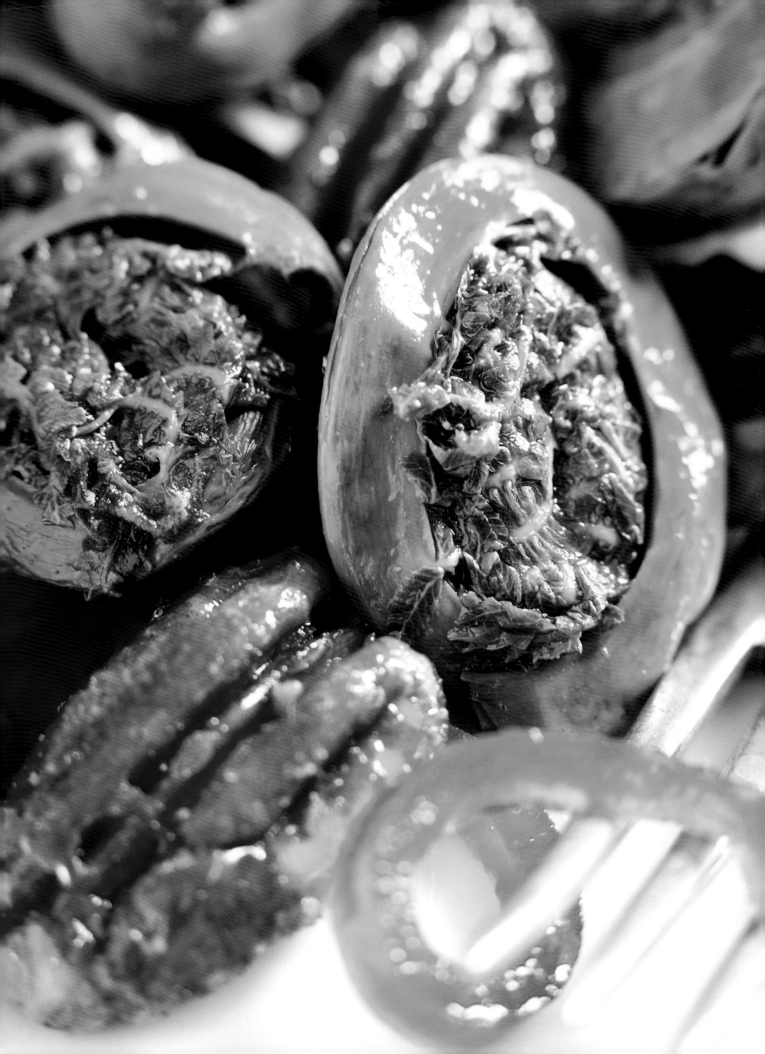

FIDDLEHEAD SALAD

Vinaigrette

3 Tbsp	lemon juice	45 mL
1 Tbsp	finely minced shallot	15 mL
½ tsp	Dijon mustard	2 mL
⅓ cup	grapeseed or canola oil	80 mL
2 Tbsp	tepid water	30 mL
	salt & pepper	
1 Tbsp	chopped chives	15 mL

Fiddleheads

3 cups	fresh or frozen fiddleheads	750 mL
3 cups	radicchio leaves (Treviso radicchio, if available)	750 mL
1 cup	pickled red onions	250 mL
⅔ cup	maple toasted pecans	160 mL

For the vinaigrette, whisk the lemon juice, shallot, and Dijon to blend. Gradually whisk in the oil until it's incorporated, then whisk in the water. Season to taste and stir in the chives.

If using fresh fiddleheads, trim off the stem ends and soak them in water for 10 minutes. Wash thoroughly, rubbing gently between your fingers. Drain well.

Bring a pot of water to a boil and salt it generously. Blanch the fiddleheads until tender, about 5 minutes for fresh and 3 minutes for frozen (tasting is the best way to judge). Drain the fiddleheads and shock them in ice water to halt the cooking process. Drain and chill until ready to serve.

To assemble the salad, arrange the radicchio on a platter. Toss the fiddleheads with the vinaigrette and arrange on the platter. Spoon the pickled red onions overtop and sprinkle with the maple toasted pecans. Serve immediately.

GOAT CHEESE TRUFFLES *Makes about 36 truffles*

Need a new idea for your cheese platter? These nibbles are easy to pick up and eat and they're not at all complicated to make.

FRESH TAKE

- One of the first signs of life to peek out of the garden, chive is a signature springtime flavor. Chives have a gentle onion nip that enhances dishes without overpowering them. Also on the spring roster of herbs: mint, tarragon, and lemon balm.

- I notice that I am using words like "mild," "delicate," and "tender" a fair bit in this chapter. My choice of words is not accidental. Spring is about new life, and in the brief growing time in the garden preceding spring harvests, robust flavors and coarse textures don't have the opportunity to develop. Keep this in mind when choosing wines to go with spring dishes. Wines described by similar adjectives suit the dishes they're accompanying: delicate Gewürztraminers, Rieslings, and Sauvignon Blancs and light Gamays and Pinot Noirs are ideal companions.

- I really like the combination of pink and green here. Pink peppercorns are quite mild (and are actually a berry, not from the pepper family at all), so even completely covered in them, the goat cheese isn't too heady.

9 oz	fresh goat cheese	270 g
6 Tbsp	finely chopped fresh chives	90 mL
6 Tbsp	finely chopped pistachios	90 mL
1½ Tbsp	finely crushed pink peppercorns mixed with 1½ Tbsp (22.5 mL) finely chopped parsley	22.5 mL

Divide the goat cheese into 2 pieces and, with damp hands, roll it into 2 long narrow logs. Cut each log into 18 pieces and shape them into balls.

Arrange the chives, pistachios, and pink peppercorn/parsley mixture each into 3 small bowls. Roll each goat cheese truffle into one of these coatings and place on a baking tray or plate. Chill until ready to serve.

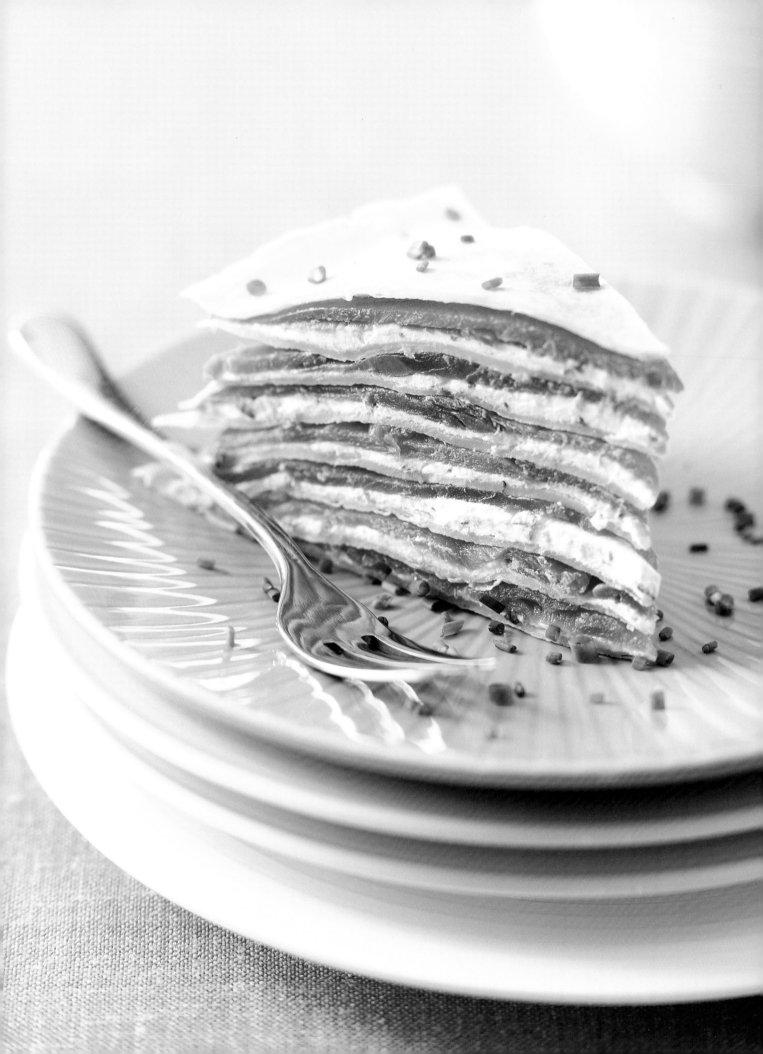

SMOKED SALMON CRÊPE TORTE

Luther Miller is a great friend and a great chef. We worked together quite a few years ago, but this creation of his has stuck with me. It's a great make-ahead hors d'oeuvre, perfect for elegant entertaining without last-minute fussing.

Just like a dessert torte, this savory version shows off thin layers in profile once sliced—of crêpe, cream cheese, and smoked salmon.

FRESH TAKE

- Beer or club soda is the secret to these crêpes. The bubbles lift the batter, and the tiny little air pockets set as the crêpe cooks, making them irresistibly tender.

- Don't feel limited to assembling the crêpes, herbed cream cheese, and salmon in just this way. Spread the cream cheese onto the crêpes, place a layer of salmon on top of each, and then roll, slicing each roll into spirals after chilling. Or make crêpe parcels filled with the salmon and cream cheese, warming them just slightly for a nice appetizer.

- When crêpes first come off the heat, they're quite delicate and tear easily. Once they've cooled completely, you'll find it easy to spread the cream cheese over them.

CRÊPES

Makes 18 small (or 12 large) crêpes

3	large eggs	3
1½ cups	2% milk	375 mL
1⅔ cups	all-purpose flour	410 mL
1 Tbsp	sugar	15 mL
¼ tsp	salt	1 mL
2 Tbsp	vegetable oil, plus more for greasing pan	30 mL
1 cup	beer or club soda	250 mL

Line a baking tray with parchment paper.

Whisk together the eggs and milk to combine and whisk in the flour, sugar, and salt. Let sit for 15 minutes (or chill until ready to use), then stir in the oil followed by the beer or club soda.

Heat a crêpe pan or other large nonstick skillet over medium heat and grease lightly. Ladle 2 to 3 Tbsp (30 to 45 mL) of batter into the center of the pan and swirl it to make a thin, even layer. Cook just until the surface of the crêpe looks dry and the edges curl up a little. Flip it over and cook for 30 seconds, then transfer it to the prepared tray to cool.

Repeat with the remaining batter. Fan the crêpes on the prepared tray (with the edges overlapping) to cool.

Once cooled, all the crêpes and wrap them in plastic wrap—no need to separate them. Store at room temperature if using them on the same day, or freeze for later use. (Do not refrigerate, however, as they will dry out.)

Continued . . .

SMOKED SALMON CRÊPE TORTE
Makes 2 small tortes •
Slices into 24 hors d'oeuvre portions

1	8 oz (225 g) pkg cream cheese, at room temperature	1
2 Tbsp	sour cream	30 mL
2 Tbsp	capers	30 mL
2 Tbsp	chopped chives	30 mL
1 tsp	finely grated lemon zest	5 mL
18	small crêpes	18
⅔ lb	(about 30 slices) good-quality smoked salmon, very thinly sliced	350 g

In a food processor, pulse the cream cheese and sour cream until smooth. Pulse in the capers, chives, and lemon zest and set the mixture aside.

To assemble, lay out 2 crêpes. Spread a thin layer of cream cheese over each and top with a single layer of smoked salmon (trim the salmon pieces if required). Place 1 crêpe on a serving plate, and top with the second crêpe. Repeat the process of layering salmon and crêpes, finishing with the ninth crêpe. Wrap the 2 "tortes" in plastic wrap and chill for at least 3 hours.

Alternatively, increase the cream cheese recipe by half, "frost" the outside of the crêpe torte, and press extra chives on the outside. (This will make it look more like a cake.) Cover and chill.

To serve, cut each torte into 12 wedges, trimming the outside edge if necessary.

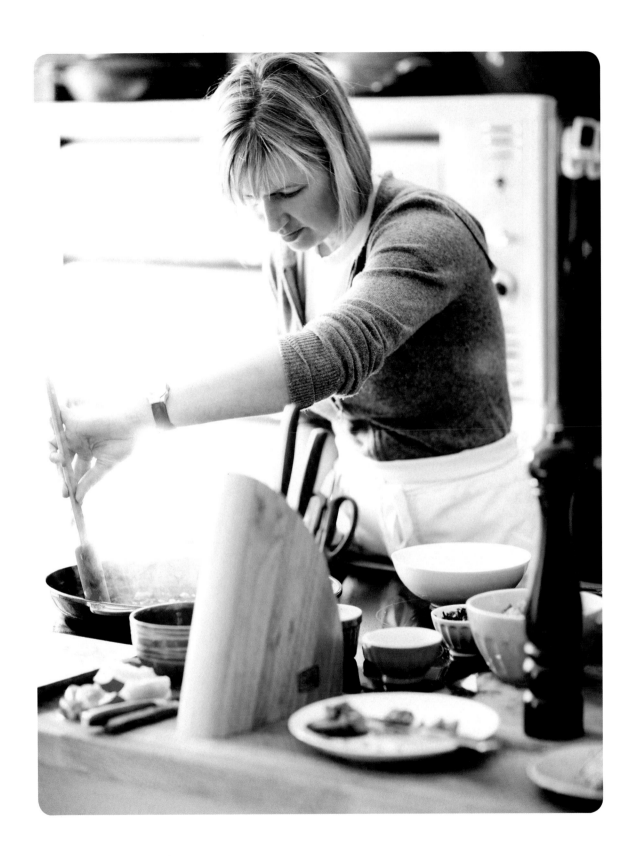

SMOKED TROUT MOUSSE on BLINIS

There seems to be a constant search for new bases for hors d'oeuvres outside of the standard crostini or cucumber slice. Blinis are a classic Russian mini pancake, originally designed to hold beluga caviar. The smoked trout mousse is far more accessible, affordable, and politically acceptable.

Hors d'Oeuvre

FRESH TAKE

- Smoked trout is altogether different from smoked salmon. Most commercial smoked salmon is cured slightly and then cold-smoked, keeping its vibrant color and soft, uncooked (though now well-preserved) texture. Smoked trout is cured but then hot-smoked (so it's fully cooked), it has a paler hue, and it flakes just like any full-cooked fish.

- Some seafood mousses are whipped, set with gelatin, and shaped in a mold. My recipe here is an easy style of mousse that is light and airy, and it can also be piped or spooned into individual ramekins or serving dishes for people to help themselves.

- Buckwheat flour and yeast set blinis apart from other pancakes. The fermentation of the yeast adds a depth of flavor that is simply magical when served with a glass of champagne or sparkling wine, and the nuttiness of the buckwheat flour complements the intensity of the smoked trout. A truly sophisticated combination.

BLINIS
Makes 5 to 6 dozen blinis

2 Tbsp + ½ cup	all-purpose flour	30 mL + 125 mL
¾ tsp	instant dry yeast	4 mL
1½ cups	2% milk, at room temperature	375 mL
2 Tbsp	buckwheat flour	30 mL
2	large eggs, separated	2
pinch	salt	pinch
2 Tbsp	whipping cream	30 mL

Stir 2 Tbsp (30 mL) of the flour, the yeast, and 1 cup (250 mL) of the milk to combine. Cover and let rest at room temperature for 20 minutes. Stir in the remaining ½ cup (125 mL) flour and the buckwheat flour, egg yolks, and salt until evenly blended. Whip the egg whites to soft peaks and set aside. Whip the cream to soft peaks and fold into the flour mixture. Fold in the whipped egg whites in 2 additions and immediately cook the blinis.

Lightly grease a griddle over medium heat. Drop the blini batter by teaspoonfuls (about 5 mL) about an inch (2.5 cm) apart onto the griddle and cook for 2 minutes. Gently flip the blinis over and cook for 1 minute more. Remove to a plate and repeat with the remaining batter. Wrap and store the blinis at room temperature until ready to serve, or freeze for up to 1 month.

SMOKED TROUT MOUSSE

Makes about 2 cups (500 ml) •
Tops 48 hors d'oeuvres

½ lb	smoked trout (or smoked salmon)	250 g
1	8 oz (225 g) pkg cream cheese, at room temperature	1
⅓ cup	whipping cream	80 mL
2 Tbsp	lemon juice	30 mL
2 Tbsp	chopped fresh chives	30 mL
1 Tbsp	chopped fresh dill (plus extra sprigs for garnish)	15 mL
½ tsp	ground black pepper	2 mL
	dill sprigs, for garnish	

In a food processor, pulse the smoked trout and cream cheese, scraping the bowl often. Add the cream and lemon juice and pulse until smooth. Scrape the mousse into a bowl and stir in the chives, dill, and pepper. Chill until ready to serve.

To assemble, pipe the mousse onto the blinis and garnish with a small dill sprig.

RICOTTA-STUFFED ZUCCHINI FLOWERS
with ROASTED PEPPER PESTO *Serves 8*

Such a delicacy! The tender blossom of the zucchini plant is just asking to be stuffed, battered, and fried. I like to use a light, tempura-style batter so as not to weigh down the blossoms. My supplier, Dave Irish, is so proud of his zucchini blossoms that he posted a photo of them on Facebook.

Double the filling if the zucchini flowers are large—3 inches (8 cm) or longer.

FRESH TAKE

- Zucchini blossoms are most common in the home vegetable garden. While some farmers' markets may offer them for a hefty price, you're not likely to find them at a major grocery store. Since zucchini are not supposed to be terribly difficult to grow (I say "supposed," as I cannot proclaim myself to be a gardener), your own garden is the best place to go shopping for these!

- Try the roasted pepper pesto on its own. Tossed with cooked pasta or served as a sauce for grilled chicken or as a dip for crudités, it satisfies that spring craving for color.

Pesto

1 cup	roasted, peeled, and sliced red bell peppers	250 mL
½ cup	lightly toasted pine nuts	125 mL
3 Tbsp	grated Parmesan	45 mL
2 Tbsp	extra virgin olive oil	30 mL
1 clove	garlic, minced	1 clove
1 tsp	finely grated lemon zest	5 mL
	salt & pepper	

Zucchini Flowers

1 cup	creamy ricotta cheese	250 mL
3 Tbsp	grated Parmesan	45 mL
3 Tbsp	chopped fresh basil	45 mL
1 clove	garlic, minced	1 clove
1 tsp	finely grated lemon zest	5 mL
	salt & pepper	
16	fresh zucchini flowers	16
	vegetable oil, for frying	

Batter

1 cup	all-purpose flour	250 mL
pinch	salt	pinch
1	egg	1
1 cup	cold soda water	250 mL
	extra flour, for dipping flowers	

For the pesto, pulse all the ingredients in a food processor until smooth (adding water if necessary) and season to taste. Chill until 1 hour before serving.

For the zucchini flowers, stir the ricotta with the Parmesan, basil, garlic, and lemon zest and season to taste. Fill a piping bag fitted with a large, plain tip with the cheese mixture. Gently wash the zucchini flowers then dry on paper towels. To fill the flowers, open them gently, trying not to tear the petals open. Remove the stamen and pipe in the filling. Chill the flowers until ready to cook.

Heat the oil in a deep pot (or tabletop deep-fryer) to 375°F (190°C).

For the batter, whisk all the ingredients together immediately before using. Sprinkle the filled flowers lightly with flour and dip them in the batter. Gently use a slotted spoon to set the flowers in the hot oil, 4 or 5 at a time, and fry for 2 to 3 minutes, turning once. Remove onto a paper towel to drain.

To serve, spoon a little pesto on a plate and arrange 2 zucchini flowers on top. Serve immediately.

BEET & GOAT CHEESE TERRINE *Makes 6 individual terrines*

The natural and subtle tartness of the goat cheese is perfectly in scale against the sweetness of the beets. With a side salad, these individual terrines make for a light lunch or a nicely sized appetizer for dinner.

Light Entrée

FRESH TAKE

- When boiling beets, be sure to leave the tops and tails on—if the beets are cut, it can leach out color as it cooks, though adding lemon to the water helps the color stay bright.

- A Japanese mandolin is an indispensable kitchen tool for a job like slicing beets thinly and consistently (it's also perfect for potatoes and other vegetables), and is found in most kitchen stores. Its blade can be adjusted to control the thickness of the cut. The finger guard is there for a reason—I highly recommend its use!

- I have to confess that I tried this recipe once with tinned beets to save time. Unfortunately tinned beets are too soft and don't slice as cleanly. Fresh is best, once again . . .

1½ lb	fresh beets	750 g
1	lemon, cut in half	1
12 oz	fresh goat cheese	375 g
2 Tbsp	whipping cream	30 mL
1 Tbsp	finely chopped chives	15 mL
1 Tbsp	finely chopped fresh mint	15 mL
1 tsp	finely grated lemon zest	5 mL
	salt & pepper	

Line 6 muffin tin cups or six 4 oz (110 mL) ramekins each with plastic wrap.

Cook the whole beets, untrimmed, in boiling water with the lemon halves until tender, about 45 minutes. Drain, discard the lemon, cool, and then peel. Slice them as thinly as possible and set aside.

Beat the goat cheese with the whipping cream until smooth. Add the remaining ingredients, season to taste, and fill a piping bag with a large, plain tip with this mixture.

To assemble, place a single beet slice in the bottom of each prepared muffin cup. Line the sides of each cup with beets, bending them gently to fit into the edge if necessary, so that each cup is entirely lined with beets. Pipe goat cheese filling into each and top the cheese with beet slices. Chill for at least 2 hours.

To serve, gently pull out each terrine, unwrap, and turn out onto a serving plate.

The terrines can be served on a bed of baby greens and a little cucumber with a simple vinaigrette. Alternatively, you can add an extra layer of smoked salmon or cooked shrimp inside or on top for a lunch entrée.

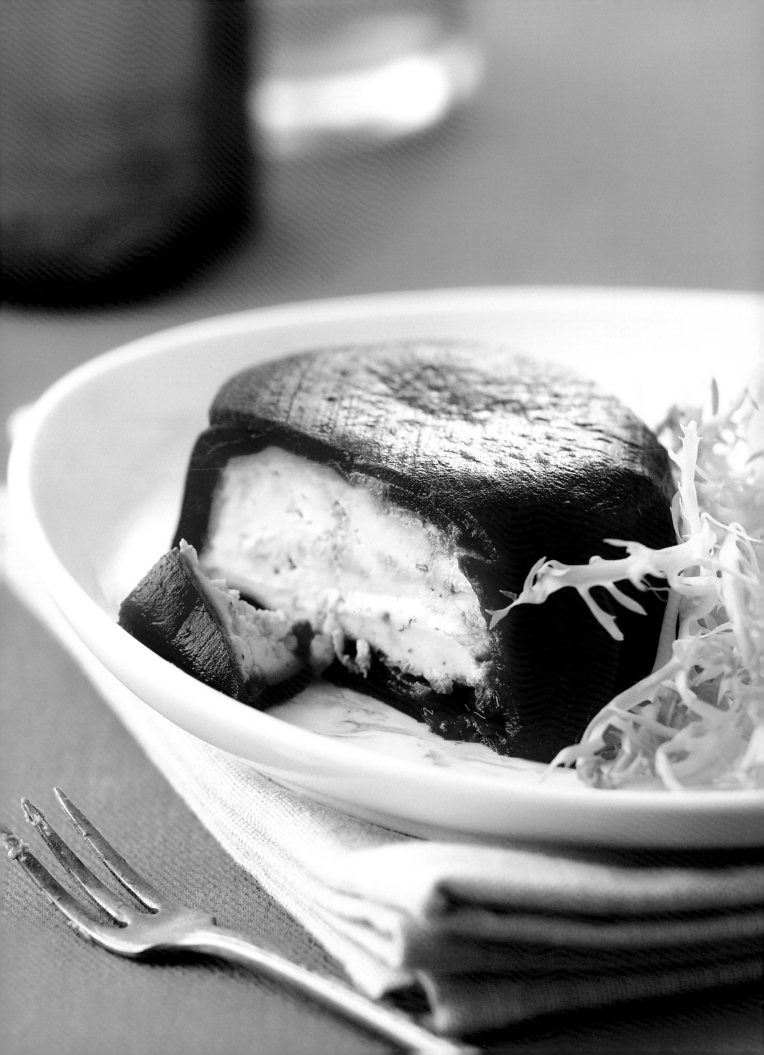

GLAZED GRILLED SALMON with
BALSAMIC ONIONS *Serves 6*

As the spring weather really starts to warm up, firing up the grill is in our thoughts. While the balsamic onions have that gooey, caramelized character of wintry dishes, the sweet zip of the balsamic wakes up our palate in time for the spring season.

FRESH TAKE

- Typically rosemary is not an herb I turn to in spring (except maybe with lamb), but when it's young, it's a fair bit milder than its fall version. I also find that salmon is one of the few fish that is enhanced by rosemary. The fattiness of salmon, particularly Atlantic salmon, suits this herb.

- I'm a big fan of a traditional barbecue sauce, but spring seems a little early to bring out my spicy-and-sweet tomato concoction. Brushing the grilling salmon with balsamic glaze accomplishes the same result, but with a little more subtlety.

- Don't bother using your special reserve balsamic vinegar for this recipe. Because of the infusing and reducing, a decent grocery-grade balsamic will do the trick.

- I grill the salmon with the barbecue uncovered, which I prefer to do for quick-cooking items and/or items grilled at high or medium-high heat. I like to cover the grill for slow-cooking foods like ribs.

Balsamic Onions

2 Tbsp	olive oil	30 mL
2	large onions, sliced	2
⅓ cup	balsamic vinegar, divided	80 mL
	salt & pepper	

Salmon

½ cup	balsamic vinegar	125 mL
2 sprigs	fresh rosemary	2 sprigs
6	4 oz (125 g) salmon fillet portions, pin bones removed	6
	olive oil	
	salt & pepper	

For the balsamic onions, heat the oil in a large sauté pan over medium heat. Sweat the onions, stirring often, until all the liquid has evaporated, about 20 minutes. Add half the balsamic vinegar and simmer until absorbed. Add the remaining balsamic and reduce to a glaze. Season to taste and set aside.

For the salmon, preheat a grill to medium-high. Reduce the balsamic with the rosemary in a small saucepot to a glaze consistency, about 8 minutes, and set aside. Brush the salmon fillets lightly with olive oil and season. Grill skin side up for 4 minutes, then rotate 90 degrees and cook for 4 more minutes to make a grid pattern. Turn the salmon over and cook for 8 more minutes for medium doneness. Brush the salmon with the balsamic glaze during the last 5 minutes of cooking.

Serve the salmon with the balsamic onions on the side.

JERK-MARINATED CHICKEN BREASTS *Serves 6*

Green, green, green! This herb paste is inspired by Jamaican jerk marinade, but without the heat of habanero peppers. Slather it over every inch of the chicken and let the sunshine in.

Poultry

FRESH TAKE

- I've based this marinade on a recipe given to me by a fellow chef I worked with in the South. Troy used to cook his mother's jerk chicken recipe for the staff meal in the kitchen before dinner service. A little chili heat can really fire you up to cook for three hundred people at a busy spot in the French Quarter.

- The combination of allspice, ginger, thyme, and oregano in a green onion base makes this distinctively "jerk" in style. And like good jerk, this rub is also fantastic on pork, fish, or shrimp.

- Some recipes (like soup) are even better the second day, and this is one of them. I love having leftovers of this chicken—they make for a great sandwich!

2 cups	chopped green onion	500 mL
2 cloves	garlic, chopped	2 cloves
3 Tbsp	chopped fresh thyme	45 mL
3 Tbsp	chopped fresh oregano	45 mL
¼ cup	extra virgin olive oil	60 mL
2 tsp	salt	10 mL
2 Tbsp	freshly grated ginger	30 mL
1½ tsp	ground allspice	7.5 mL
1½ tsp	ground black pepper	7.5 mL
½ tsp	ground nutmeg	2 mL
	chili flakes or ground chili pepper, if desired (to taste)	
6	boneless, skinless chicken breasts	6
	lime juice, for sprinkling	

In a food processor, or with a mortar and pestle, purée the green onion, garlic, thyme, and oregano with the olive oil and salt until finely processed. Stir in the ginger, allspice, black pepper, nutmeg, and chili (if using).

Coat the chicken breasts with the herb mixture, cover, and chill for at least 30 minutes to a maximum of 24 hours.

Preheat the oven to 375°F (190°C). Line a baking tray with parchment paper.

Place the chicken breasts on the prepared baking tray, being sure to spoon any excess herb mixture on top, and roast them, uncovered, until cooked through and the juices run clear when cut, about 25 minutes. Slice and serve warm or at room temperature, sprinkled with lime juice.

Alternatively, the chicken can be grilled over medium heat, turning once during cooking, about 25 minutes.

ONION-MARINATED SIRLOIN with SPICY SPRING SALSA *Serves 6*

What an unexpected and fabulous combination! No prissy strawberry dish, this chili-spiked salsa is a great companion to grilled beef, especially if served rare to medium-rare.

FRESH TAKE

- Puréeing the onion to rub over every inch of the beef ensures maximum contact and flavor. Once grilled, the remaining onion covering the beef also cooks, even caramelizing in spots, so it never tastes too strongly.

- When I make strawberry desserts, such as the Strawberry Meringue Tarts (page 38), I like to let the cut berries sit to draw out the juices. The little bit of sugar and salt help this along, and then, once the juices have reduced, the intensity of the fruit increases.

- This salsa is a fantastic way to use up very ripe berries—you can cut away any soft bits (bruised berries lose their sweetness) and use up berries that might have become compost in a day or so.

3 cups	roughly chopped onion	750 mL
3 cloves	garlic, chopped	3 cloves
3 Tbsp	white wine vinegar	45 mL
2 Tbsp	Dijon mustard	30 mL
1 Tbsp	ground black pepper	15 mL
3 Tbsp	extra virgin olive oil	45 mL
5 lb	top sirloin steak, about 2 inches (5 cm) thick	2.2 kg
	coarse salt	

In a food processor, pulse the onion, garlic, vinegar, mustard, and pepper until smooth. Drizzle in the oil while the processor is running, and pour the marinade into a large, shallow dish. Place the sirloin in the dish and then turn to coat it with the marinade. Cover and chill for at least 4 hours to a maximum of 24 hours, turning occasionally.

Preheat the grill to medium heat.

Remove all but a thin layer of the marinade from the beef and season with salt. Place on the grill and cover. Grill on 1 side for about 12 minutes, rotating it 90 degrees once to make crisscrossing grill marks, then turn and grill it on the other side for about the same time for medium-rare (use a temperature probe and grill the steak to an internal temperature of 135°F/57°C). Let the sirloin rest for 5 minutes before slicing.

Any leftover marinade can be brought to a boil then simmered for 5 minutes, then served on the side as a relish beside the spring salsa (or toss it into a side dish of boiled potatoes).

Makes about 2 cups (500 ml)

2 cups	diced fresh strawberries	500 mL
½ cup	chopped green onion	125 mL
3 Tbsp	white balsamic or rice wine vinegar	45 mL
pinch	sugar	pinch
pinch	salt	pinch
1 tsp	chopped fresh tarragon	5 mL
½ tsp	chili flakes	2 mL

Toss the strawberries and green onion with the white balsamic, sugar, and salt, and let them sit for 30 minutes. Strain off the liquid that comes out into a small pot and simmer it until it has a glaze consistency. Add the glaze to the strawberries and stir in the tarragon and chili flakes. Taste for seasoning and chill until ready to serve.

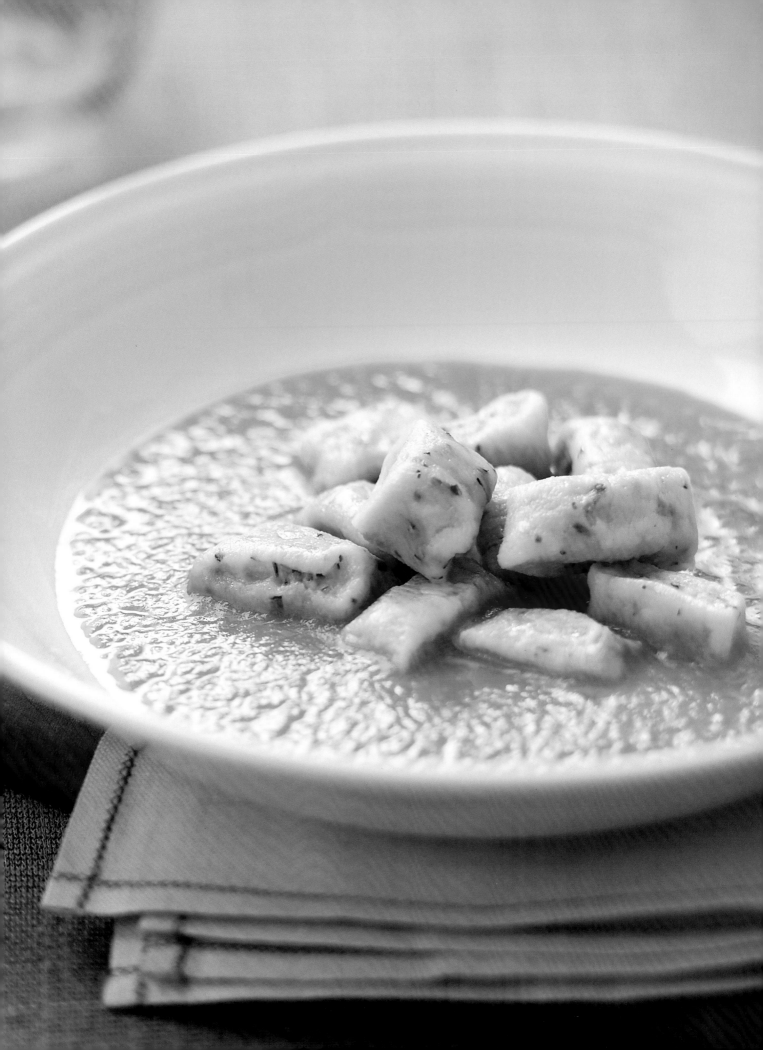

GOAT CHEESE GNOCCHI with
PEPPER COULIS *Serves 6*

Potato gnocchi are filling and satisfying in winter, and fluffy ricotta gnocchi are pleasant in summer, so it follows that these gnocchi are the perfect dish to bridge the two extremes. Served in a bright, fresh-tasting sauce, this is truly a taste of spring.

FRESH TAKE

- Regardless of where you live, early to late spring is peak season for hothouse produce. Buying local hothouse peppers, tomatoes, and cukes is a perfect way to shop locally and enjoy great-tasting produce after a long winter.

- When handling and rolling out the gnocchi dough, feel free to generously flour your work surface and hands—these gnocchi will still remain soft and fluffy. The dough is delicate but not fragile, moist but not too sticky either. Once you cook them and taste your first one, you'll see what I mean!

- This pepper sauce is simple and bright. If you don't want to use wine, simply substitute the same measure of water plus 1 Tbsp (15 mL) lemon juice in its place.

Pepper Coulis

¼ cup	olive oil	60 mL
1 cup	diced onion	250 mL
2½ cups	diced red bell pepper	625 mL
¾ cup	dry white wine	185 mL
2 sprigs	fresh thyme	2 sprigs
2 sprigs	fresh oregano	2 sprigs
	salt & pepper	

Goat Cheese Gnocchi

4 oz	fresh goat cheese, at room temperature	125 g
4 oz	cream cheese, at room temperature	125 g
3 Tbsp	finely chopped green onion	45 mL
2 Tbsp	finely chopped flat-leaf parsley	30 mL
1 Tbsp	finely grated lemon zest	15 mL
2	eggs, separated	2
1 cup	all-purpose flour	250 mL
½ tsp	salt	2 mL

For the pepper coulis, heat the oil in a saucepot over medium heat. Sauté the onion for 5 minutes, until translucent. Add the peppers and sauté for 3 minutes more. Add the wine and herbs and simmer, covered, until the peppers are tender, about 10 minutes. Remove from the heat and purée. Strain, season, and set aside.

For the gnocchi, beat the goat cheese and cream cheese until smooth. Stir in the green onion, parsley, lemon zest, and egg yolks until smooth. Fold in the flour. Whip the egg whites with the salt to soft peaks and fold into the goat cheese mixture in 2 additions.

Bring 16 cups (4 L) water to a boil and salt generously. Cut the dough in half. Roll out 1 piece into a log shape about ¾-inch (2 cm) in diameter and cut it into ½-inch (1 cm) pieces. Place on a floured tray and repeat with the second piece of dough. Drop the gnocchi into the water in 2 batches and simmer until they float, about 3 minutes. Gently remove with a slotted spoon. To serve, heat the coulis and spoon it into a flat-bottomed bowl. Gently place gnocchi on top.

Starch

HOMEMADE TORTELLINI with FENNEL CREAM *Serves 4 to 6*

I'm a big fan of filled pasta like ravioli and this classic Tuscan tortellini. Even served in a cream sauce, this dish is not terribly heavy.

FRESH TAKE

- I chat with my neighbors regularly about food, and with one in particular about Italian food. She makes tortellini all the time (so I wanted to compare notes), and although she grew up making it with that distinctive addition of cinnamon in the filling, she now goes without because her kids don't like it. Try it first with, and let your own family be the judge. Personally, I like the cinnamon.

- When you're making a filled pasta like this, or something like Gyoza (page 142), an extra set of hands makes it more fun, and much less daunting. The tortellini also freeze well uncooked in an airtight container for up to two months, so stock up! Now that's fantastic convenient food.

- A little confession—I'm not one to reach for fennel for a salad; I much prefer it cooked, like in this sauce. I find the licorice tastes mellows and the texture smoothes out nicely.

Dough

2 cups + 6 Tbsp	all-purpose flour	590 mL
3	large eggs, at room temperature	3
¼ tsp	salt	1 mL

Filling

1 Tbsp	olive oil	15 mL
1 tsp	fennel seeds	5 mL
10 oz	ground pork	300 g
1¼ cups	finely grated Parmesan	310 mL
1 tsp	finely chopped fresh rosemary	5 mL
⅛ tsp	ground cinnamon	0.5 mL
⅛ tsp	ground nutmeg	0.5 mL
⅛ tsp	ground black pepper	0.5 mL
2	large eggs	2

Fennel Cream

2 Tbsp	olive oil	30 mL
1	medium onion, sliced	1
1 head	fresh fennel, thinly sliced	1 head
2 tsp	finely chopped thyme	10 mL
1 tsp	fennel seed	5 mL
½ cup	dry white wine	125 mL
2 cups	whipping cream	500 mL
	salt & pepper	
	grated Parmesan	

For the pasta dough, pulse the ingredients in a food processor until blended (the dough will be dry). Wrap it in plastic wrap and let rest refrigerated for 1 hour.

While the dough is resting, prepare the filling. Heat a medium sauté pan over medium heat and add the olive oil. Stir in the fennel seeds and toast them in the oil for 1 minute. Add the pork and cook it through. Remove the pork from the pan then toss it in a bowl with the Parmesan, rosemary, cinnamon, nutmeg, and pepper. (No need to add salt; the

Continued . . .

Starch

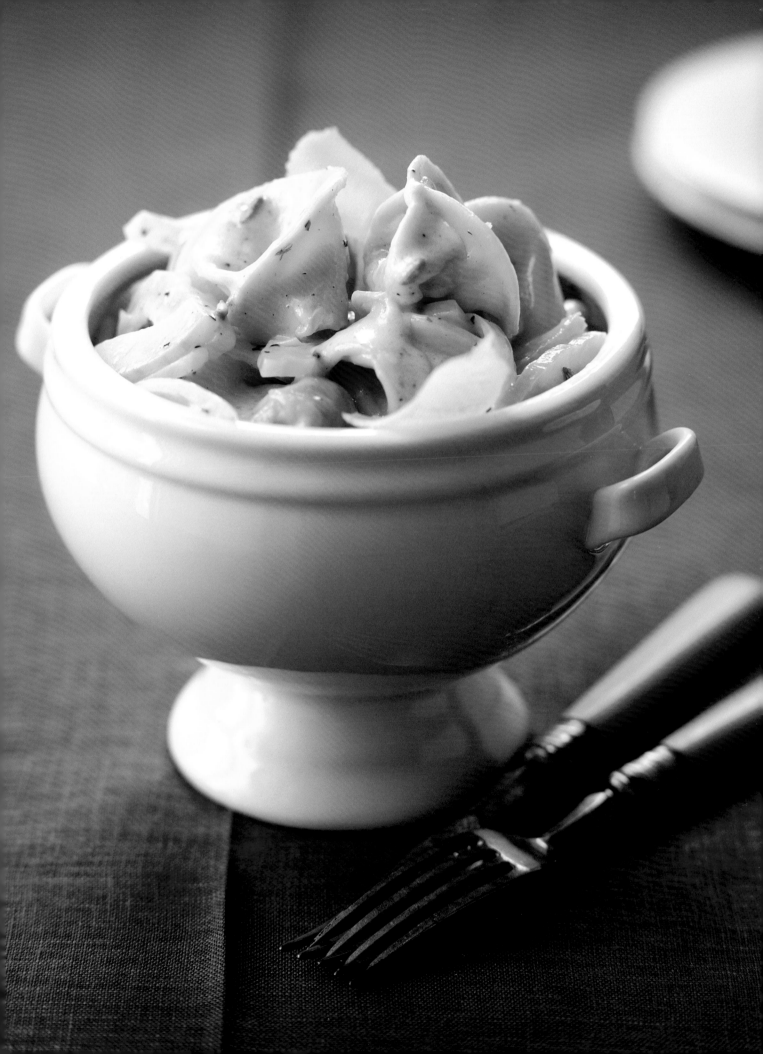

Parmesan adds sufficient salt for this recipe.) Whisk the eggs in a small bowl and stir them into the pork mixture.

Roll out the dough through a pasta machine, following the manufacturer's instructions. Cut out rounds about 2 inches (5 cm) across and spoon a teaspoonful (about 5 mL) of filling into each. Fold each circle in half and wrap around a finger, pinching the ends together to create tortellini. Set them on a baking tray and chill, uncovered, until ready to cook.

To cook the tortellini, bring a pot of water to a boil and salt generously. Add the tortellini and boil until they float, about 3 minutes. Drain well and reserve while preparing the sauce.

For the fennel cream sauce, heat the olive oil in a large sauté pan over medium heat. Add the onion and fennel and sauté until the onion is translucent, about 5 minutes. Add the thyme and fennel seed, then add the white wine and simmer until the wine is reduced by half. Add the cream and simmer until sauce consistency (it should coat the back of a spoon). Season to taste. Add the cooked tortellini, return to a simmer to warm it through, and serve garnished with Parmesan.

GREEN BEAN GRIDDLE CAKES *Makes 12 small griddle cakes*

Need an interesting way to serve green beans? I like these for family-style suppers, when you're passing around great platters of food.

FRESH TAKE

- Like making pancakes in the morning, you can make these griddle cakes a bit ahead of time and keep them covered and warm in a 250°F (120°C) oven.

- It's convenient to buy frozen frenched green beans, but it's really quite easy to cut the beans on a bias. I french the beans in the recipe so that they shape easily within the griddle cake. The technique itself is a way to make large, late-season green beans more tender by cutting into the fiber of the tougher bean.

- Michael has a weakness for yellow wax beans from the market. We only buy them when they're in season, so we don't get any stringy surprises from string beans that earn their name.

1 lb	fresh green and yellow beans	500 g
1 Tbsp	olive oil, for the batter	15 mL
½ cup	finely diced onion	125 mL
2	large eggs, separated	2
¼ cup	all-purpose flour	60 mL
½ tsp	fine sea salt	2 mL
¼ tsp	baking powder	1 mL
pinch	ground nutmeg	dash
2 Tbsp	olive oil, for the griddle	30 mL

Trim and french (slice thinly on an angle) the beans. Bring a pot of water to a boil, add salt, and blanch the beans, uncovered, until just tender, about 4 to 5 minutes. Drain and rinse to cool (or shock them in ice water). (Alternatively, you can use 2 cups (500 mL) thawed frozen frenched beans.) Set aside in a large bowl.

Heat 1 Tbsp (15 mL) of the olive oil in a small sauté pan over medium heat and sauté the onion until tender. Cool the onions slightly, add to the beans, and toss. Stir in the egg yolks, flour, salt, baking powder, and nutmeg and stir to coat the beans. In a separate bowl, whip the egg whites until they hold a soft peak, and fold into the batter in 2 additions.

Heat a griddle over medium heat with the remaining 2 Tbsp (30 mL) olive oil and drop the batter by spoonfuls onto the griddle, cooking for about 3 minutes. Flip the griddle cakes over gently and cook for 3 minutes more. Repeat with remaining batter until all griddle cakes are made.

Serve with butter or a small dollop of sour cream.

Vegetables

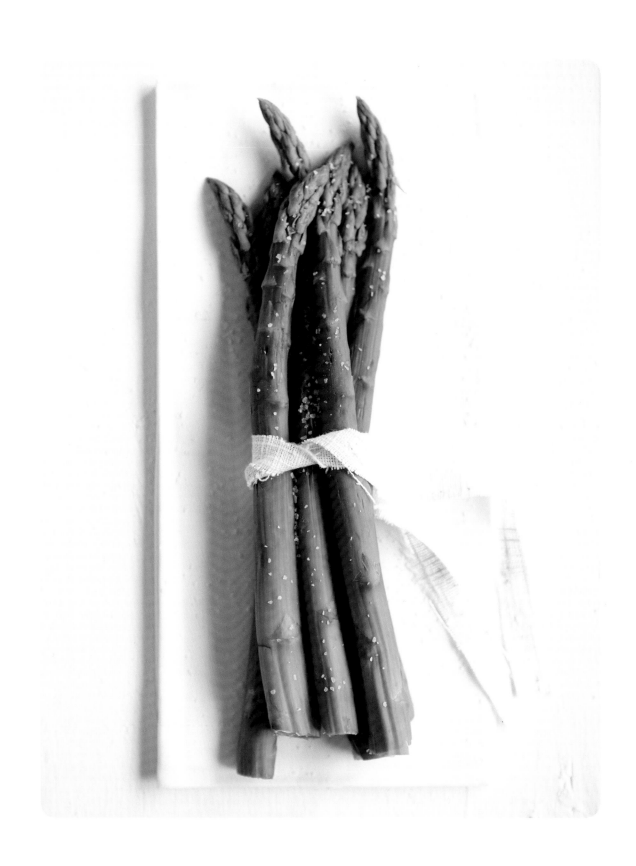

ASPARAGUS with RHUBARB HOLLANDAISE

Serves 6

I have a weakness for a good hollandaise, especially when it's served with asparagus in season. At the same time, rhubarb comes into its own, and its fruity acidity replaces a traditional wine or vinegar base for this warm, buttery sauce.

FRESH TAKE

- If blanching asparagus in boiling water (versus steaming), it's important to boil it uncovered so that it retains its bright green color. And by shocking it with ice water, you halt the cooking and the green color will set, even when reheated.

- The principle behind a hollandaise is to gently cook the egg yolks so that they don't scramble. The acidity in the lemon juice helps prevent curdling while the yolks hit their appropriate temperature. To be certain, you can always use a thermometer to check that the mixture reaches 160°F (71°C).

- Michael turned me onto this delightful springtime combination of rhubarb and asparagus. This dish used to be on the menu at Inn on the Twenty, a wine-country restaurant in the Niagara, when we worked there together. See, it's okay to take work home with you sometimes!

2 lb	fresh asparagus	1 kg

Rhubarb Hollandaise

1¼ cups	finely diced fresh or frozen rhubarb	310 mL
⅓ cup	sugar	80 mL
2 sprigs	fresh tarragon	2 sprigs
2	large egg yolks	2
3 Tbsp	lemon juice	45 mL
½ cup	melted butter	125 mL
	salt & pepper	

To Finish

	butter, for sauté pan	
	chopped chives, for garnish	

Bring a pot of water to a boil and salt generously. Trim the asparagus and blanch, uncovered, until tender (check by tasting as the time will vary depending on its thickness). Once tender, drain then shock the asparagus in a bowl with ice and water to halt the cooking process. Strain and chill the asparagus until ready to serve.

For the hollandaise, stir the rhubarb, sugar, and tarragon sprigs in a pot over medium heat. Simmer until the rhubarb is just tender, about 10 minutes. Remove the tarragon and keep the rhubarb warm (but not hot).

Whisk the egg yolks and lemon juice in a bowl over a pot of gently simmering water (making sure the bowl's not touching) until the yolks hold a ribbon when the whisk is lifted. Whisk in the rhubarb mixture to warm slightly. Remove the bowl from the heat and gradually whisk in the melted butter (try to avoid adding any white solids that have settled at the bottom of the butter). Season to taste and keep warm (hollandaise should be prepared as close to serving as possible).

To heat the asparagus, simply warm it in a sauté pan over medium-low heat with butter and season lightly. Place the warm asparagus on a platter and spoon hollandaise overtop. Garnish with chives and serve immediately.

CITRUS HARICOTS VERTS *Serves 4*

Two bean recipes in one section? Well, of course! When it's in season, you just gotta cook it. With any variety, whether green, yellow, or dainty haricots verts, the key is to relish every bite, because before you know it the season has passed and you have to wait until next year to enjoy it at its best.

FRESH TAKE

- *Haricots verts* simply translates to "green beans." Our interpretation has taken on a little further meaning, referring to a variety that is very small, slender, and tender. We should really call them "haricots petits," shouldn't we?

- I like to serve this alongside other French flavors, like the Turkey Escalope (page 108). And the citrus garnishes make this a wine-friendly companion, for either a crisp dry Riesling, which typically has citrus notes, or a buttery Chardonnay.

- You have to serve these beans immediately after you add the citrus and finish the sauce—as they sit the acidity in the orange and grapefruit will turn them brown. *Pas bien!*

1 lb	fresh small green beans, washed	500 g
2 Tbsp	olive oil	30 mL
1 clove	garlic, minced	1 clove
1 tsp	finely grated orange zest	5 mL
⅔ cup	water	160 mL
1	navel orange, segmented without membrane	1
1	red grapefruit, segmented without membrane	1
1 tsp	sugar	5 mL
2 Tbsp	cold butter	30 mL
	salt & pepper	

Trim the ends from the beans. Heat the olive oil in a large sauté pan over medium-high heat. Add the beans and toss to coat. Add the garlic and orange zest and sauté for 1 minute. Add the water and simmer the beans, uncovered, until almost all the water has evaporated, about 4 minutes. Transfer the beans to a serving dish. Add the orange and grapefruit segments to the pan and stir gently to warm them through, just until the juices come out. When they begin to simmer, stir in the sugar and remove the pan from the heat. Stir in the cold butter in small pieces until it's melted. Season to taste and spoon over the beans.

HAM & SCALLION SCONES with LEMON-HERB CHÈVRE *Makes 16 to 20 small scones*

While some reach for a gooey sticky bun or an extra helping of maple syrup over their pancakes in the morning, others reach for something more savory.

These scones are as nice alongside a cup of tea in the afternoon as they are with scrambled eggs in the morning. The lemon chèvre makes a refreshing change from cream cheese or butter.

FRESH TAKE

- I like to work in the butter with my fingers, not just with a pastry cutter. This way I connect with the dough, and can better feel the texture of it. While a scone dough is not as delicate as a pie dough, it's important to have little pieces of butter still present before you add the buttermilk so that the scone bakes up flaky and tender.

- Fresh goat cheese has an inherent citrus taste to it, so it suits a little enhancement by way of added lemon. Use this anywhere you like to use flavored cream cheese—on a toasted bagel with smoked salmon, on crostini alongside a bowl of soup, or with crackers and pepper jelly.

- I'm one of those people who prefer a cookie or something sweet with the afternoon cup of tea, but I like something savory to start my day if oatmeal (my favorite) isn't on the menu. When I'm at the bakery, I'm more apt to grab a roll and a slice of ham and cheese than to reach for a muffin.

3 cups	all-purpose flour	750 mL
¼ cup	sugar	60 mL
1 Tbsp	baking powder	15 mL
½ tsp	salt	2 mL
¾ cup	cold unsalted butter	185 mL
1 cup	buttermilk, plus extra for brushing	250 mL
1 cup	diced Black Forest ham, cut into ½-inch (1 cm) pieces	250 mL
1 cup	chopped scallions (green onions)	250 mL

Preheat the oven to 375°F (190°C). Line a baking tray with parchment paper.

In a large bowl, stir the flour, sugar, baking powder, and salt to blend. Cut in the butter with a pastry cutter or 2 knives until you have a rough, crumbly texture. (I favor this method over a mixer or food processor. You may also use your fingers to work in the butter.) Stir in the buttermilk, ham, and scallions. Once combined, turn the dough onto a work surface. Using your hand, flatten and fold the dough a few times, incorporating the dry crumbs at the same time, until you can shape it into a disk. Press or roll the dough flat to about ¾ inch (2 cm) thick and use a 2-inch (5 cm) cutter to cut out scones, rerolling and cutting until all the dough has been used. Arrange the scones on the prepared baking tray. Brush the scone tops with more buttermilk and bake for about 17 minutes, until a rich, golden color. Serve warm or at room temperature.

Scones are best served the day they're baked, but baked scones, as well as the dough, freeze well. Simply thaw the dough for 6 hours in the fridge before baking.

Continued . . .

LEMON-HERB CHÈVRE
Makes 1 cup (250 ml)

6 oz	fresh goat cheese (chèvre)	175 g
1 tsp	finely grated lemon zest	5 mL
2 Tbsp	lemon juice	30 mL
2 Tbsp	sour cream or buttermilk	30 mL
2 Tbsp	finely chopped fresh dill	30 mL
1 Tbsp	finely chopped fresh mint	15 mL
	salt & pepper	

Beat the chèvre, lemon zest and juice, and sour cream or buttermilk until fluffy. Stir in the herbs, season to taste, and chill, covered, until ready to serve.

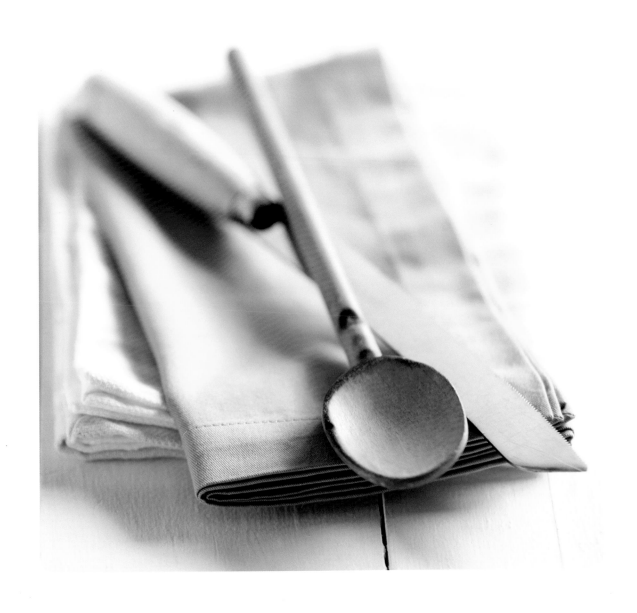

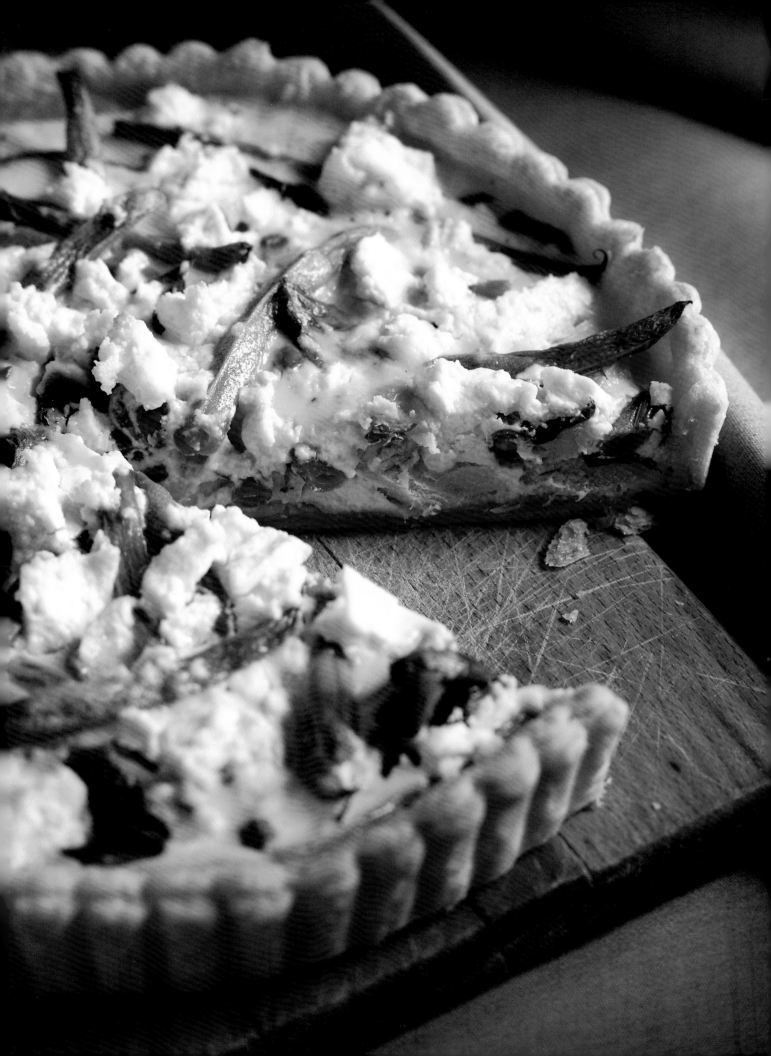

PEAMEAL, GREEN BEAN, & CHEESE TART

Makes one 9-inch (23 cm) tart • Serves 6 to 8

Quiche may be a breakfast and brunch staple, but I find it benefits from a little makeover now and again. This fluted tart has an elegant presentation, and is a step up from quiche Lorraine.

FRESH TAKE

· The Parmesan tart crust is tasty and tender, but when it chills overnight it can become very firm. It's important to chill the dough, though, so that it's easier to roll and the glutens (proteins) relax for a tender crust that doesn't shrink. If you make the dough a day ahead, you need to pull it out from the fridge about 90 minutes before you roll it so it handles a little easier.

· I like the salty kick that the capers lend to this tart, but they could be easily replaced by pitted, chopped kalamata olives.

· A thin slice of this tart would also make a nice hors d'oeuvre or appetizer alongside a salad of spring greens. A few tender pea shoots dressed with a little olive oil make a perfect springtime companion.

· This tart can be made a day ahead, chilled, and reheated in a 325°F (160°C) oven for 30 minutes.

Crust

1½ cups	all-purpose flour	375 mL
½ cup	cold unsalted butter, cut into pieces	125 mL
⅓ cup	finely grated Parmesan	80 mL
¼ cup	cold water	60 mL

Filling

¼ lb	peameal bacon, cooked	125 g
¼ lb	green beans, trimmed and blanched	125 g
⅓ cup	loosely packed fresh basil leaves	80 mL
1 Tbsp	capers	15 mL
2	eggs + 1 egg yolk	2
¾ cup	sour cream	185 mL
¼ tsp	salt	1 mL
¼ tsp	black pepper	1 mL
2½ oz	fresh goat cheese	75 g

For the crust, pulse the flour and butter in a food processor until they have a rough, crumbly texture. Add the Parmesan and water and pulse until the dough comes together. Turn the dough out, shape it into a disk, wrap, and chill until firm but not hard, about 30 minutes.

Preheat the oven to 375°F (190°C). On a lightly floured surface, roll out the dough to a circle just less than ¼ inch (6 mm) thick. Line an ungreased 9-inch (23 cm) removable-bottom tart shell with the dough, trimming the edges. Chill for 30 minutes. Line the tart shell with parchment paper or tinfoil and fill with dried beans, raw rice, or pie weights. Bake for 15 minutes, lift off the paper or tinfoil, and bake another 15 minutes until golden. Let it cool.

Reduce the oven temperature to 350°F (180°C). Julienne the peameal bacon and sprinkle over the bottom of the crust. Arrange the green beans over the bacon, tear the basil and sprinkle overtop, then finish off with the capers.

In a small bowl, whisk the eggs, egg yolk, sour cream, salt and pepper. Carefully pour this over the tart fillings and crumble goat cheese overtop. Bake on a baking tray for about 30 minutes, until the eggs are set but don't soufflé at the edges. Cool for 15 minutes before slicing.

STRAWBERRY MERINGUE TARTS *Makes 6 individual tarts*

Elegant and feminine, these tarts are fully "tarted up." While the casual dollop of meringue on each tart reminds me of a generous helping of whipped cream, it is a light-as-air meringue that sweetens up the fresh berry filling.

FRESH TAKE

- Ripe berries can let out a lot of juice the moment you slice them. I was inspired to create this berry filling so as not to waste a drop. The juices, thickened with cornstarch, hold the berries in place. This tart keeps a fresh strawberry taste, as opposed to a cooked pie filling.

- This tart shell recipe has a shortbread-like buttery goodness but enough structure to hold up to the fresh berry filling without going soggy.

- It only takes two minutes for the heat of the hot oven to permeate the meringue right to the center and cook it. Don't go too far from the oven or you'll have a toasted-marshmallow strawberry tart.

Crust

1¼ cups	pastry flour, sifted	310 mL
1½ Tbsp	sugar	22.5 mL
¼ tsp	salt	1 mL
6 Tbsp	cold unsalted butter, cut into pieces	90 mL
1	egg yolk	1
½ tsp	white vinegar	2 mL
3 Tbsp	cold water	45 mL

Filling

3 cups	quartered fresh strawberries	750 mL
1 cup	sugar	250 mL
1 Tbsp	lemon juice	15 mL
½ cup + 2 Tbsp	water	125 mL + 30 mL
3 Tbsp	cornstarch	45 mL

Meringue

5	large egg whites	5
1 tsp	lemon juice	5 mL
½ cup	sugar	125 mL
1 tsp	cornstarch	5 mL

For the crust, blend the flour, sugar, and salt in a mixer fitted with a paddle attachment. Cut in the butter, on low speed, until a rough crumbly texture. In a separate bowl, whisk the egg yolk with the vinegar and cold water. Add this all at once to the flour mixture and blend. If the dough is still crumbly, add 1 to 2 Tbsp (15 to 30 mL) water. Shape the dough into a log, wrap in plastic wrap, and chill for at least 1 hour.

Divide the dough into 6 equal pieces. On a lightly floured surface, roll out each piece of dough to just less than ¼ inch (6 mm) thick, and line six 3½-inch (9 cm) tart shells with dough. Trim the tart shells and chill for 30 minutes to 1 hour.

Preheat the oven to 350°F (180°C).

Place the tart shells on a baking tray and dock the bottoms with a fork. Bake for 15 to 18 minutes, until the bottoms appear dry and the edges are lightly browned. Let cool.

Continued . . .

Sweets

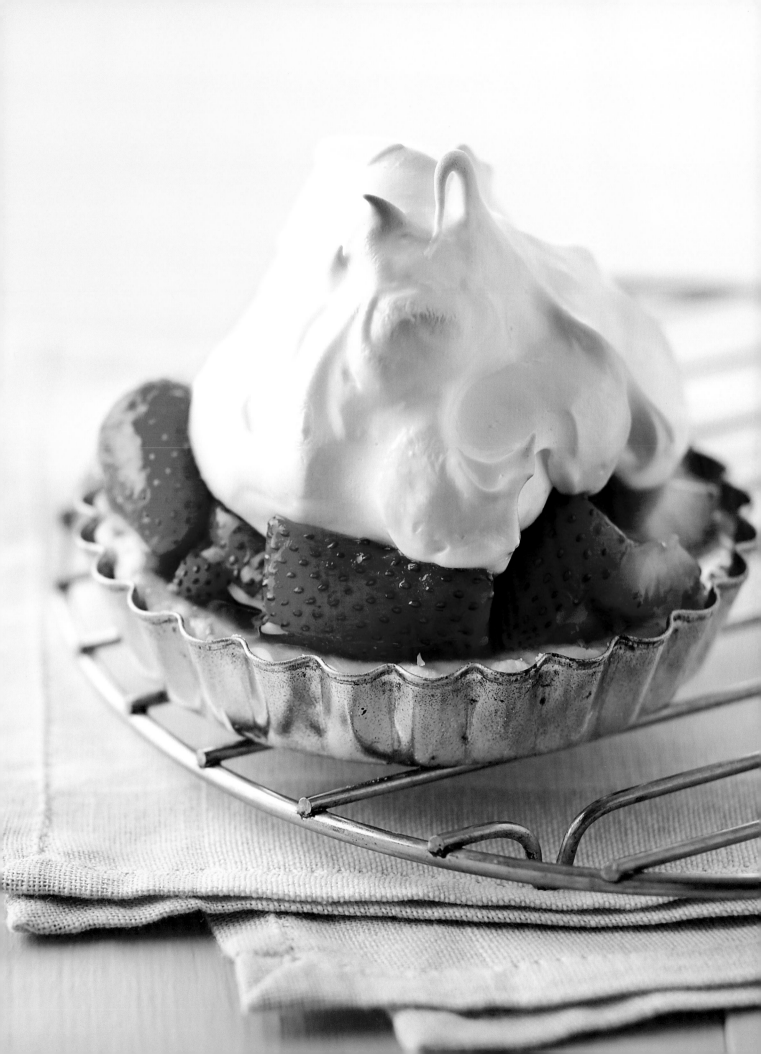

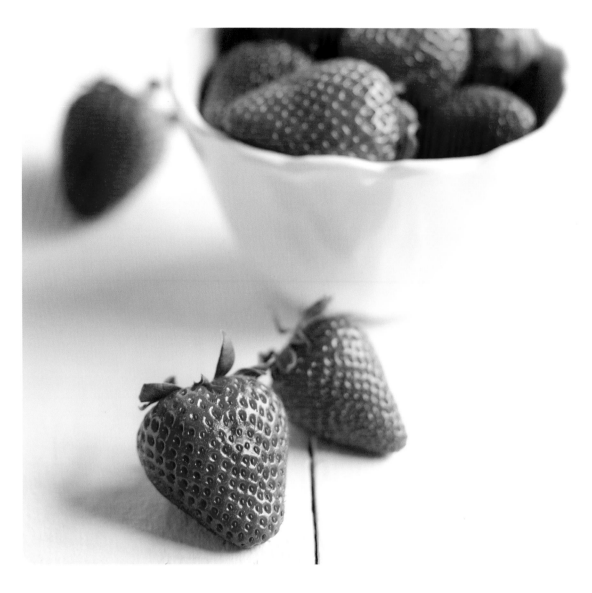

Strawberry Meringue Tarts (continued)

For the filling, stir the strawberries with the sugar, lemon juice, and ½ cup (125 mL) water. Let them sit for 20 minutes. Strain the liquid into a small pot and bring it to a simmer. Stir the cornstarch with 2 Tbsp (30 mL) water and whisk it into the simmering liquid. Stir until the filling has thickened, then remove the pot from the heat to cool. Once cooled, fold the sauce into the strawberries and spoon them into the baked tart shells. Chill the tarts while preparing the meringue.

Preheat the oven to 400°F (200°C).

Whip the egg whites with the lemon juice on one speed lower than high and gradually add the sugar while whipping to stiff peaks. Stir in the cornstarch then pipe or dollop the meringue over the strawberry filling. Bake for 2 to 3 minutes until browned, then cool and chill until ready to serve.

HONEY YOGURT "CHEESECAKE"

Makes one 9-inch (23 cm) dessert • Serves 8

Yes, you can make a low-fat cheesecake that's dense and delicious! A combination of drained yogurt and ricotta cheese bakes into a tangy cheesecake that will convert you into a low-fat cheesecake lover.

FRESH TAKE

- Draining yogurt to use in place of fresh cheese is not a new technique but it is easy. Sweetened with a little honey, yogurt cheese can also replace whipped cream as a dolloped garnish on fresh fruit or any cake or tart.

- While it's just fine to use low-fat ricotta in this recipe, it's ideal to use regular, full-fat yogurt for the cheesecake. Regular yogurt strains better and keeps its body when baked, while low- or nonfat versions turn to liquid.

- Sweetening desserts with honey takes a delicate hand—honey has a distinctive taste, floral and unique, and in larger amounts can taste even sweeter than sugar. It's amazing how only ¼ cup (60 mL) of honey (not very much!) sweetens and flavors this whole dessert perfectly.

Yogurt "Cheese"

2 cups	3.5% yogurt	500 mL
2 cups	creamy ricotta cheese (low-fat is fine)	500 mL

Crust

2 cups	graham cracker crumbs	500 mL
1 tsp	finely grated lemon zest	5 mL
¼ tsp	salt	1 mL
½ cup	unsalted butter, melted	125 mL

Filling

1 recipe	yogurt cheese	1 recipe
¼ cup	honey	60 mL
1	egg	1
1 tsp	finely grated lemon zest	5 mL
1 tsp	vanilla extract	5 mL

Topping

1½ cups	diced fresh mango, strawberries, or other fresh fruit	375 mL

Prepare the yogurt "cheese" a day before needed. Stir the yogurt and ricotta together and place in a cheesecloth (or large paper coffee filter) set inside a strainer. Place the strainer over a bowl, cover loosely with plastic wrap, and chill for 24 hours. Discard the whey (the liquid in the bowl) and refrigerate the yogurt cheese until ready to use.

Preheat the oven to 325°F (160°C).

For the crust, combine the graham cracker crumbs, lemon zest, salt, and melted butter and press the mixture into an ungreased 9-inch (23 cm) pie plate. Bake for 10 minutes, then cool while preparing the filling.

For the filling, stir the yogurt cheese with the honey, egg, lemon zest, and vanilla. Spoon this into the cooled crust and bake for 30 minutes. Cool to room temperature then chill for at least 4 hours before serving.

Top with diced mango, strawberries, or other fresh fruit immediately before slicing.

INDIVIDUAL CRÈME BRÛLÉE CHEESECAKES

Makes 6 cheesecakes

Two of our favorite desserts combined into one decadent treat. Because these are served individually, no one can argue that they got a smaller portion.

Cheesecakes

1	1 lb (500 g) tub good-quality mascarpone cheese	1
½ cup	sugar	125 mL
½ cup	whipping cream	125 mL
1 Tbsp	vanilla bean paste OR scraped seeds from 1 vanilla bean	15 mL
3	large eggs	3

Phyllo Wafers

3 sheets	phyllo pastry	3 sheets
¼ cup	unsalted butter, melted	60 mL
2 Tbsp	sugar (plus extra for "brûlée")	30 mL

Preheat the oven to 325°F (160°C). Grease six 5 oz (150 mL) ramekins and place a disk of parchment in the bottom of each. Place the ramekins in a baking dish with a 2-inch (5 cm) lip.

For the cheesecakes, stir the mascarpone gently to soften it. Add the sugar and combine well. Stir in the whipping cream and vanilla bean paste (or vanilla bean seeds), switching to a whisk to smooth out the mixture. Whisk in the eggs one at a time until blended. Ladle the mixture into the prepared ramekins and pour hot tap water in the baking dish to halfway up the ramekins. Bake the cheesecakes for 35 minutes (the tops of the cheesecake will brown to golden), then remove them from the water bath to cool. Chill for at least 6 hours before serving.

Increase the oven temperature to 350°F (180°C). Line a baking tray with parchment.

For the phyllo wafers, lay out 1 sheet of phyllo. Brush it lightly with butter and sprinkle with sugar. Cover with a second sheet of phyllo and brush with butter and sprinkle with sugar again. Repeat with a third sheet, then fold the phyllo layers in half. Cut 6 circles out of the pastry with a 3½-inch (9 cm) cookie cutter and place them on the prepared baking tray. Bake for 7 minutes, until golden brown. Let cool.

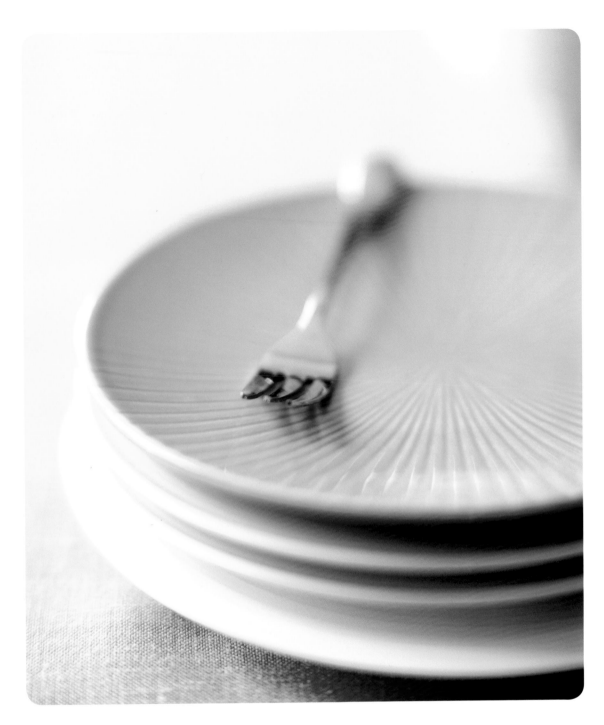

To serve, place a phyllo wafer on a dessert plate. Run a spatula around the inside of each ramekin to loosen the cheesecake then turn it out onto each wafer. Peel away the parchment disk and sprinkle sugar over the top of the cheesecake. Using a kitchen butane torch (available at kitchen supply stores), caramelize the top of the cheesecake. Repeat with the remaining cheesecakes and serve.

SUMMERTIME

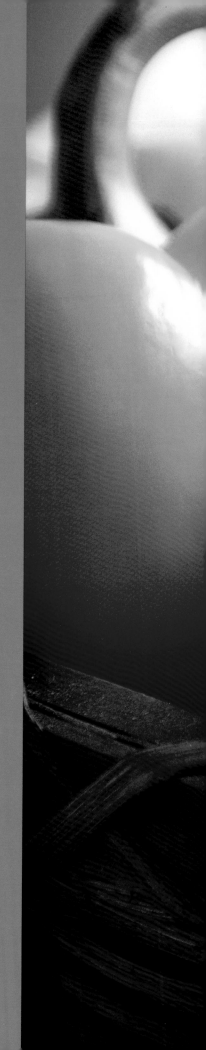

The first thing that comes up when I think of summertime isn't a sight, a smell, or even a taste. It's a sound—the hum of cicadas on the hottest day, which makes you slow your pace to little more than a crawl. (I don't have air conditioning at home, so every sound on the street is integrated into my day-to-day activities.)

And the farmers' markets are bursting with everything imaginable. I always buy far too much. In July and August, I drive by no fewer than six farm-gate stands where growers put out their offerings on a card table and ask for payment on the honor system. Too often, after a trip to the farmers' market or past these farm gates, Michael and I have so much fresh produce to contend with that we put away the chicken or steak we pulled out and just make a meal out of vegetables.

We also tend to eat later in the evening, making a full day out of activities, and light the grill as the sun starts to set. I love eating on our porch, as the dusk seems to linger for an eternity. Many of the dishes I prepare for summer suppers are fine served at room temperature, so we can take our time and eat slowly, in the hopes that, if we take our time, summer will last just a little bit longer.

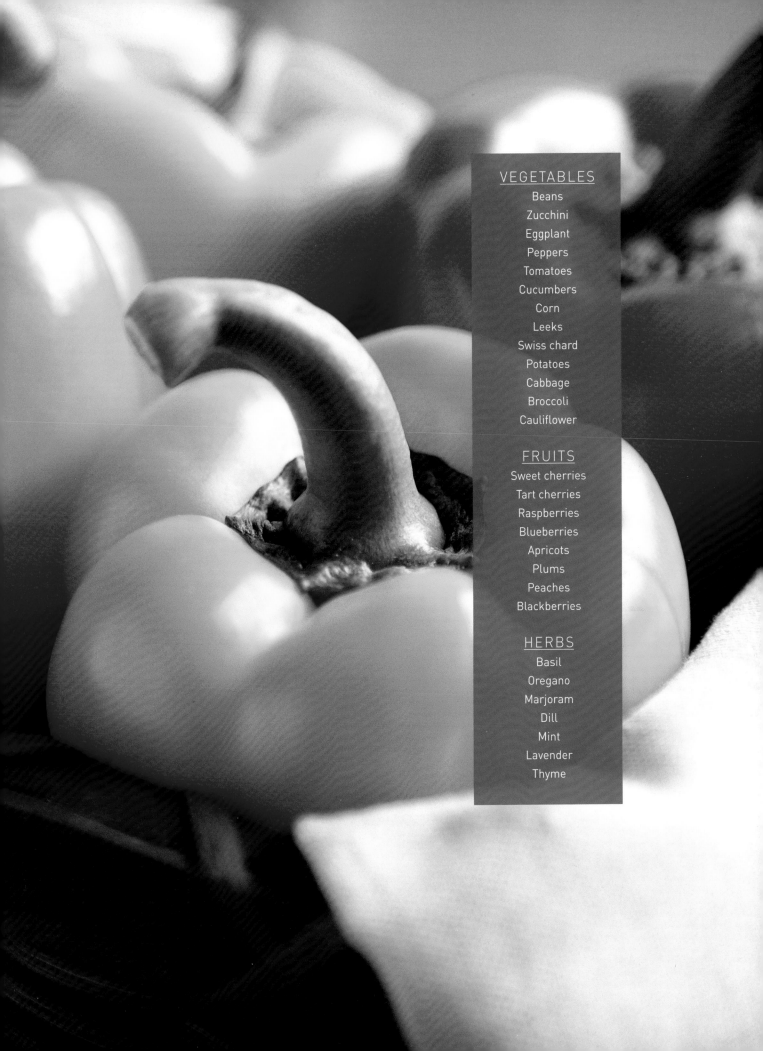

VEGETABLES
Beans
Zucchini
Eggplant
Peppers
Tomatoes
Cucumbers
Corn
Leeks
Swiss chard
Potatoes
Cabbage
Broccoli
Cauliflower

FRUITS
Sweet cherries
Tart cherries
Raspberries
Blueberries
Apricots
Plums
Peaches
Blackberries

HERBS
Basil
Oregano
Marjoram
Dill
Mint
Lavender
Thyme

RIBOLLITA (TUSCAN VEGETABLE SOUP)

Serves 6 to 8

This soup adds to the belief that soup is always better the second day, and lends credence to its Italian translation, "reboiled." A hearty vegetable concoction is ladled over day-old bread, chilled, and then baked to reheat the next day. The bread soaks up some of the broth, so this soup can be a meal in itself.

FRESH TAKE

- Cabbage is one of those vegetables that changes its identity between summer and winter. Because it stores well, it pops up on dinner plates in winter, usually thoroughly braised, soft, and melting. But in summer, cabbage is fresh and biting, appearing alongside our grilled burgers as coleslaw. In this soup, it really sits in the middle—it cooks until tender, but not as soft as its winter self.

- A smoked ham hock is a secret weapon in soup making. It yields only a little meat but loads of flavor when cooked into a broth. The smokiness rounds out all the other flavors as the soup cooks.

- I have yet to visit Tuscany (sigh), but I spend a great deal of time reading about it and looking online for rentals. A small part of me is almost afraid to visit. After hearing so many wonderful tales from friends and family who have made the journey, I'm afraid that I might have built up the region in my mind so much that I will only be disappointed when I arrive. Well, there's only one way to find out!

3 Tbsp	olive oil	45 mL
4 strips	thick-sliced bacon, diced	4 strips
2 stalks	celery, diced	2 stalks
2	medium carrots, peeled and diced	2
1	small leek, white and light green parts only, thinly sliced	1
1	medium onion, diced	1
2 cloves	garlic, minced	2 cloves
8 cups	chicken stock	2 L
3 sprigs	fresh thyme	3 sprigs
1	smoked ham hock	1
3 cups	shredded Savoy cabbage	750 mL
2	14 oz (398 mL) cans navy beans, drained and rinsed	2
	salt & pepper	
3 cups	diced day-old white bread, cut into ½-inch (1 cm) cubes	750 mL

Heat a heavy-bottomed soup pot over medium heat and add the olive oil and bacon. Cook the bacon until crisp, remove it from the pan, and drain all but 2 Tbsp (30 mL) of the fat. Add the celery, carrots, leek, and onion and sauté until the onion is translucent, about 5 minutes. Add the garlic and sauté for 1 minute more. Add the stock, thyme, and ham hock and bring to a simmer. Cover the pot and simmer for 45 minutes. Add the cabbage and simmer for 15 minutes more. Purée 1 can of the navy beans with 1 cup (250 mL) of the soup liquid then add it back to the soup. Add the remaining can of beans to the soup. Remove the ham hock to cool. Season to taste.

Lay the bread cubes in a deep baking or casserole dish. Shred the meat from the ham hock and sprinkle it over the bread. Ladle the soup over the bread and let it cool. Chill the soup overnight.

Preheat the oven to 375°F (190°C).

Cover the soup dish and heat until the soup is bubbling at the edges, about 40 minutes. Serve immediately.

TENDER GREEN SALAD with GRILLED APRICOTS & RED ONION VINAIGRETTE *Serves 6*

I like to serve this salad with my Marinated Flank Steak (both pictured on page 66), with the vinaigrette drizzled not only over the salad greens but over the steak, too.

FRESH TAKE

- This vinaigrette is a summer staple in our house. Toss it with shredded cabbage for instant coleslaw, or drizzle it over ripe tomatoes topped with crumbled blue cheese.

- Apricots have such a brief season, you have to enjoy them while you can get them. If the season misses you (or you miss the season), you can substitute peaches instead for this recipe.

- To toast the walnut pieces, it's best to spread them on an ungreased or parchment-lined baking tray and toast them for 12 minutes in a 350°F (180°C) oven, stirring once. If it's just too hot to turn on the oven, toast them in a sauté pan placed on the grill, tossing often until the fragrance of the toasted nuts wafts up.

Red Onion Vinaigrette

⅓ cup	chopped red onion	80 mL
3 Tbsp	red wine vinegar	45 mL
2 tsp	honey	10 mL
1 tsp	finely chopped fresh tarragon	5 mL
1 tsp	Dijon mustard	5 mL
¾ cup	canola or grapeseed oil	185 mL
	salt & pepper	

Salad

6	fresh apricots, cut in half and pitted	6
6 cups	mixed tender greens, such as Boston or leaf lettuce	1.5 L
½ cup	lightly toasted walnut pieces	125 mL
⅓ cup	crumbled feta cheese	80 mL

For the vinaigrette, pulse the onion, vinegar, honey, tarragon, and mustard in a food processor or with a handheld blender until smooth. While blending, slowly pour in the oil until incorporated. If the vinaigrette is too thick, whisk in 2 to 3 Tbsp (30 to 45 mL) warm water. Season to taste.

To build the salad, grill the apricot halves over high heat, turning them once just to soften them and add grill marks, about 4 minutes. Slice the apricot halves in half again and toss them with 2 Tbsp (30 mL) of the vinaigrette. Arrange the salad greens on a platter and arrange the apricots on top. Sprinkle the salad with walnut pieces and feta and dress immediately before serving (or serve the vinaigrette on the side).

GRILLED PEPPER & EGGPLANT SALAD *Serves 8*

Instead of the predictable basil and garlic combination, I pair garlic accents with those of orange, sesame, and ginger, which makes this a tasty companion to any grilled fish or meat, or a hearty addition to an antipasti platter.

FRESH TAKE

· I prefer not to brush my eggplant with oil before I grill it. Eggplant is porous and will soak up as much oil as you give it. Since it won't stick to the grill (provided the grill is clean), I prefer to dress the eggplant after cooking.

· I find this salad is best served at room temperature because of the intensity of the accent flavors. If you serve it chilled, the orange, ginger, and garlic will be merely an aftertaste since they'll wake up after they hit your warm palate, sadly just a little too late. Serving this at room temperature ensures a balanced and well-timed melding of the flavors.

· This is a salad that embraces spice, if the mood should strike. Stir in a seeded and minced jalapeño pepper or chili flakes, or a sprinkle of your favorite hot sauce, for a kick.

1	medium eggplant, sliced lengthwise into ½-inch (1 cm) slices	1
2	red bell peppers, cut into quarters, stem and seeds removed	2
	juice and zest of 1 orange	
1 clove	garlic, minced	1 clove
1 Tbsp	toasted sesame seeds	15 mL
2 tsp	finely grated fresh ginger	10 mL
3 Tbsp	olive oil	45 mL
	salt & pepper	
2 Tbsp	chopped flat-leaf parsley	30 mL

Preheat the grill to medium-high heat, or preheat the oven to 400°F (200°C) and line a baking tray with parchment paper.

If you're grilling, cook the eggplant slices and pepper quarters (without brushing with oil) until lightly charred, but still moderately firm, turning them occasionally. Remove them from the heat into a bowl and cover with plastic (this will continue to soften the vegetables).

If you're oven-roasting, place the eggplant and peppers on the prepared baking tray and roast for 15 minutes, turning them once. Remove the vegetables from the tray into a bowl and cover with plastic.

Once the vegetables have cooled for about 10 minutes, slice them into bite-sized pieces. (No need to remove the skins from the peppers.) Toss with the orange juice and zest, garlic, sesame seeds, ginger, and olive oil. Season to taste and spoon them into a serving dish. Sprinkle parsley overtop and keep in the fridge.

Bring the salad to room temperature before serving.

TENDER GREENS with MARINATED SWEET CHERRIES in ALMOND VINAIGRETTE *Serves 6*

This refined salad makes my mouth water. Cherries and almonds are a common pairing in the dessert world, so it follows that they are well partnered in the savory world as well.

FRESH TAKE

- Like apricot season, sweet cherry season is fleeting. Sweet cherries are difficult to bake with and are usually eaten fresh, but macerating them in red wine vinegar really draws out their full potential. Ripe plums are a good replacement.

- A delicate salad such as this makes a great first course, or it can be served alongside grilled halibut or shrimp for a summer supper *alfresco*.

- Almond oil can be purchased at some grocery stores and at specialty food stores. It is more perishable than olive or canola oil, so is typically sold in a can. Store it in a cool place, or even chilled, for about 6 months to ensure its freshness. If it's difficult to locate, use a mild extra virgin olive oil.

Cherries

2 cups	pitted sweet cherries	500 mL
2 Tbsp	minced red onion	30 mL
1½ Tbsp	red wine vinegar	22.5 mL
1 Tbsp	honey	15 mL
1 Tbsp	chopped fresh mint	15 mL
pinch	ground cinnamon	pinch

Vinaigrette

2 Tbsp	red wine vinegar (optional, to replace juice from marinated cherries)	30 mL
1 tsp	honey	5 mL
1 tsp	Dijon mustard	5 mL
6 Tbsp	almond oil	90 mL
1 Tbsp	chopped chives	15 mL
	salt & pepper	

Greens

6 cups	tender greens, such as Boston, baby leaf lettuce, or even spinach	1.5 L
½ cup	lightly toasted sliced almonds	125 mL

For the cherries, toss all the ingredients together and let sit for 30 minutes to 3 hours.

For the vinaigrette, strain off 2 Tbsp (30 mL) of the cherry liquid (or use red wine vinegar) and whisk in the honey and mustard. Whisk in the oil gradually until the vinaigrette is smooth and creamy. Stir in the chopped chives and season to taste.

Arrange the tender greens on a platter. Drizzle with vinaigrette and top with marinated cherries. Sprinkle with the toasted almonds and serve.

CORN & SHRIMP FRITTERS with CUCUMBER REMOULADE
Makes about 24 fritters • Serves 6

These easy nibbles are convenient to make for a dinner party as they can actually be fried ahead and warmed in the oven for serving. Served with a remoulade sauce (a French and also Southern U.S. version of tartar sauce), it's impossible to eat just one. (Pictured on page 146.)

FRESH TAKE

- My version of remoulade is more like a garlic-free version of tzatziki with flair. Remoulade is usually mayonnaise-based, but the yogurt I use here makes this version refreshingly tangy.

- To make the fritters ahead of time, chill them after deep-frying. When it's time to serve, warm the fritters on a baking tray in a 375°F (190°C) oven for 10 minutes, then serve immediately.

- My inspiration for the fritters? New Orleans hush puppies!

Cucumber Remoulade

1 cup	finely grated cucumber	250 mL
1 tsp	sugar	5 mL
½ tsp	fine sea salt	2 mL
1 cup	yogurt	250 mL
2 Tbsp	capers, drained and chopped	30 mL
2 Tbsp	chopped dill pickle (or dill pickle relish)	30 mL

Fritters

1 Tbsp	olive oil	15 mL
½ cup	finely diced onion	125 mL
¾ cup	fresh or frozen corn kernels	185 mL
1 tsp	finely chopped fresh thyme	5 mL
1 cup	cornmeal	250 mL
½ cup	all-purpose flour	125 mL
1 Tbsp	sugar	15 mL
1 Tbsp	baking powder	15 mL
¾ tsp	salt	4 mL
pinch	black pepper	pinch
1	egg	1
¾ cup	2% milk	185 mL
1½ cups	cooked baby shrimp or salad shrimp (thawed and drained if frozen)	375 mL
	vegetable oil, for deep-frying	

For the remoulade, stir together the cucumber, sugar, and salt and place it in a strainer over a bowl for 30 minutes. Squeeze out any excess liquid, stir in the yogurt, capers, and dill pickle, and chill until ready to serve.

For the fritters, heat the oil in a small sauté pan over medium heat and add the onion. Sauté for 5 minutes until translucent, then add the corn and thyme and sauté until the corn is tender, about 3 minutes. Remove from the heat to cool.

Stir together the cornmeal, flour, sugar, baking powder, salt, and pepper. In a separate bowl, whisk together the egg

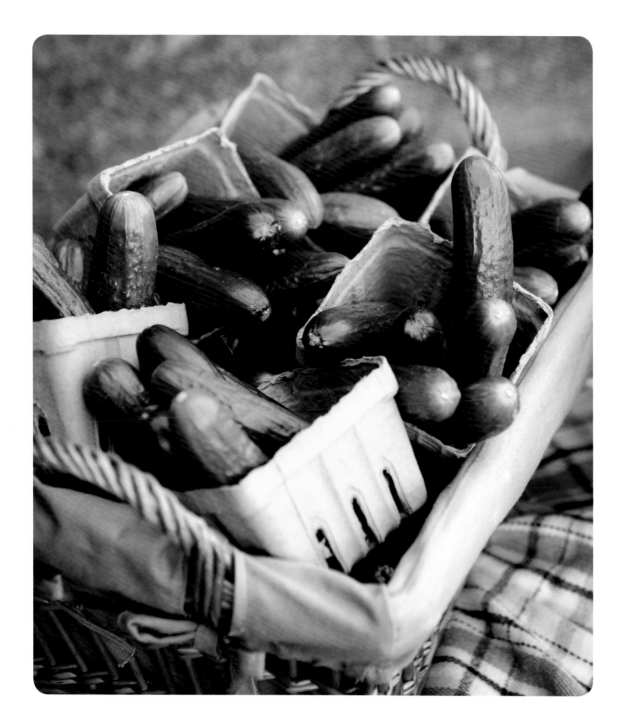

and milk. Add this to the flour mixture and stir just until blended. Fold in the cooled corn mixture, then stir in the shrimp.

Heat enough oil to come up 2 inches (5 cm) in a heavy-bottomed deep pot to 375°F (190°C). Drop the fritter batter by tablespoonfuls (about 30 mL) gently into the oil and fry until deep golden brown, turning once (about 6 minutes). Remove the fritters and place on paper towels to drain the oil. Serve warm with the remoulade. Cooked fritters can be kept warm, uncovered, in a 250°F (120°C) oven.

CORNBREAD MUFFINS with BABY SHRIMP SALAD *Makes 3 dozen mini muffins*

Just like the Corn & Shrimp Fritters (previous page), the cornbread and shrimp combination here works just perfectly for summer entertaining.

FRESH TAKE

- I made these shrimp for my friend and fellow pastry chef Andrea's baby shower. The entire theme of the shower was "baby-sized bites," hence the baby shrimp.

- Matane shrimp are small shrimp from the eastern part of Quebec, from the mouth of the St. Lawrence River. Any variety of small shrimp, known as "salad shrimp," will do.

- I like how the creaminess of the avocado, worked into the shrimp salad, binds it together and replaces any need for mayonnaise.

CORNBREAD MUFFINS

1 cup	cornmeal	250 mL
1 cup	all-purpose flour	250 mL
¼ cup	sugar	60 mL
1 Tbsp	baking powder	15 mL
½ tsp	celery salt	2 mL
1 Tbsp	chopped chives	15 mL
1 Tbsp	chopped fresh cilantro	15 mL
1 cup	buttermilk	250 mL
1	egg	1
5 Tbsp	vegetable oil	75 mL
½ cup	fresh or frozen corn kernels	125 mL

Preheat the oven to 375°F (190°C) and grease three 12-cup mini muffin tins (36 cups).

Sift the cornmeal, flour, sugar, baking powder, and celery salt into a bowl. Stir in the chives and cilantro. In a separate bowl, whisk together the buttermilk, egg, and oil. Add this to the dry ingredients, stirring just until incorporated (do not overmix). Quickly stir in the corn. Divide the batter equally among the prepared muffin cups. Bake the muffins until a tester inserted into the center comes out clean, about 8 minutes. Cool for 10 minutes, then turn out to cool completely.

BABY SHRIMP SALAD

Makes about 3 cups (750 ml)

1 ear	corn-on-the-cob, husk removed	1 ear
1¼ cups	finely diced avocado (about 1)	310 mL
1½ Tbsp	fresh lime juice	22.5 mL
3 Tbsp	finely minced red onion	45 mL
1½ lb	frozen cooked Matane baby shrimp, thawed and chopped	750 g
2 Tbsp	chopped fresh cilantro	30 mL
	salt & pepper	

Preheat the grill to high.

Grill the corn until charred lightly on all sides and the kernels are bright yellow. Let cool and transfer the kernels to a bowl.

Toss with the remaining ingredients and season to taste. The creaminess of the avocado will bind the salad together.

To serve, cut the top from each muffin and spoon a little shrimp salad inside. Cap with the muffin top if desired.

DEVILLED EGGS *Makes 16 portions*

I have a soft spot for devilled eggs, and I know I'm not alone. Whenever I put out a plate of these pretty eggs at a party, even alongside other tasty morsels, they're the first to disappear.

FRESH TAKE

· The easiest way to blend the egg yolks smoothly into the mayonnaise is to rub them through a mesh strainer— you won't have a single lump.

· Of course, using good Dijon mustard in lieu of dry mustard is just fine for this recipe. I think I use dry mustard because that's what my mom used to use, and I have to admit, it has its own particular nip.

· I find that letting the eggs sit in the water to cool is the key to a perfectly cooked egg. This method cooks the yolk all the way through without overcooking the white of the egg, and there's no greenish outer layer to the yolk.

8	eggs	8
½ cup	mayonnaise	125 mL
1½ tsp	dry mustard	7.5 mL
1 Tbsp	finely chopped fresh chives	15 mL
2 tsp	capers, drained and chopped	10 mL
	salt & pepper	
	capers and chives, for garnish	

Place the eggs in tepid water and bring up to a simmer. Cook for 4 minutes, shut off the heat, and let the eggs sit in the water until it cools to room temperature.

Peel the eggs and cut them in half. Scoop out the cooked yolks, blend them with the mayonnaise, mustard, chives, and chopped capers and season to taste. Place the egg filling in a piping bag (no tip needed for this one) and pipe it back into the egg whites. Garnish with a caper and a sprig of chive. Cover and chill until ready to serve.

POTATO & PROSCIUTTO KEBABS with GREEN GODDESS DIPPING SAUCE

Makes 8 large kebabs • Serves 8

These are hearty nibbles that can be taken to the beach to warm up over an open fire. Not so adventurous? A grill on the back deck gives the same effect.

FRESH TAKE

- I've always been a fan of Green Goddess dressing. It was created in the 1920s in San Francisco in tribute to a play (and later movie) of the same name. I appreciate this dressing, which is like a second cousin to ranch dressing, for its bright green color and herbaceous taste. (Its low oil content is a winning feature, too.)

- While I normally favor prosciutto sliced so thinly that I can read a newspaper through it, this is one occasion where slightly thicker slices work in your favor, as they make it easier to weave around the potatoes on the skewers.

- You can also use this technique with coins of zucchini, whole mushrooms, and slices of bell pepper, if you wish. Mmmm. Or you could even make an entrée skewer by adding cubed chicken or beef.

Green Goddess Dipping Sauce

1 cup	mayonnaise	250 mL
⅔ cup	chopped flat-leaf parsley	160 mL
½ cup	buttermilk	125 mL
½ cup	chopped green onion	125 mL
½ cup	loosely packed fresh basil leaves	125 mL
½ cup	loosely packed fresh mint leaves	125 mL
1 Tbsp	Dijon mustard	15 mL
3 Tbsp	olive oil	45 mL
	salt & pepper	

Kebabs

8	sturdy bamboo or metal skewers	8
2 lb	red mini potatoes (about 24 potatoes)	1 kg
1 cup	diced red onion, cut into 1½-inch (4 cm) pieces	250 mL
8 slices	prosciutto, sliced lengthwise in half	8 slices
	olive oil, for brushing	
	salt & pepper	

For the dipping sauce, purée all the ingredients, except the oil, until smooth. Slowly pour in the oil while blending and season to taste.

For the kebabs, soak the bamboo skewers (if using) in water while preparing the other ingredients. Boil the potatoes, uncovered, in salted water until tender, about 12 minutes. Drain and let them cool to room temperature.

Slice the potatoes in half (or leave them whole if small). First skewer an onion piece, then skewer the end of a prosciutto slice near the top of the skewer. Skewer a piece of potato and onion, then wrap the prosciutto tightly along 1 side of the potato and onion before skewering again. Skewer another potato and onion piece and then the prosciutto again—it will eventually create a lovely scalloped effect. Continue, using a second slice of prosciutto, until the skewer is full.

To heat, lightly brush the kebabs with oil and season. On a hot grill or over an open fire, grill until warmed through, about 6 minutes. Serve warm with dipping sauce.

CHILLED GRILLED SEAFOOD SALAD *Serves 10*

This salad makes another great addition to an antipasti platter, or as a luncheon entrée over mixed greens.

FRESH TAKE

- This is a seafood lover's dream! The lime juice and radicchio work together to bring out the inherent sweetness in the shrimp, calamari, and scallops.

- Sometimes buying frozen seafood is even better than purchasing fresh, especially if you live more than a hundred kilometers from the ocean. Often seafood is caught, cleaned, and then flash-frozen right on the ship. The key is to pat dry any thawed seafood with a paper towel before grilling so it doesn't stick to the grill.

- I picked up a great trick from my good friend Lisa for grilling without using too much oil. Simply fold up a clean kitchen towel and hold it with a pair of tongs. Dip the towel in a little vegetable oil then rub it on the clean, hot grill. It adds just enough oil to prevent sticking, but not so much that you get flare-ups.

1 lb	whole calamari, cleaned, plus tentacles	500 g
1 lb	shrimp (20/25), peeled and deveined	500 g
1 lb	large sea scallops (dry-pack frozen is okay)	500 g
1 cup	shredded radicchio	250 mL
½ cup	diced tomato	125 mL
½ cup	chopped green onion	125 mL
3 Tbsp	chopped fresh cilantro	45 mL
2 Tbsp	chopped fresh mint	30 mL
2 Tbsp	fresh lime juice	30 mL
3 Tbsp	extra virgin olive oil	45 mL
dash	hot sauce (optional)	dash
	salt & pepper	

Heat the grill to high and grill the calamari, shrimp, and sea scallops for about 3 minutes on each side (turning once). Remove from the heat and let cool.

Once the seafood is cool, cut it into bite-sized pieces. Toss with the remaining ingredients, season to taste, and chill. If preparing this more than 2 hours ahead of time, add the radicchio just before serving.

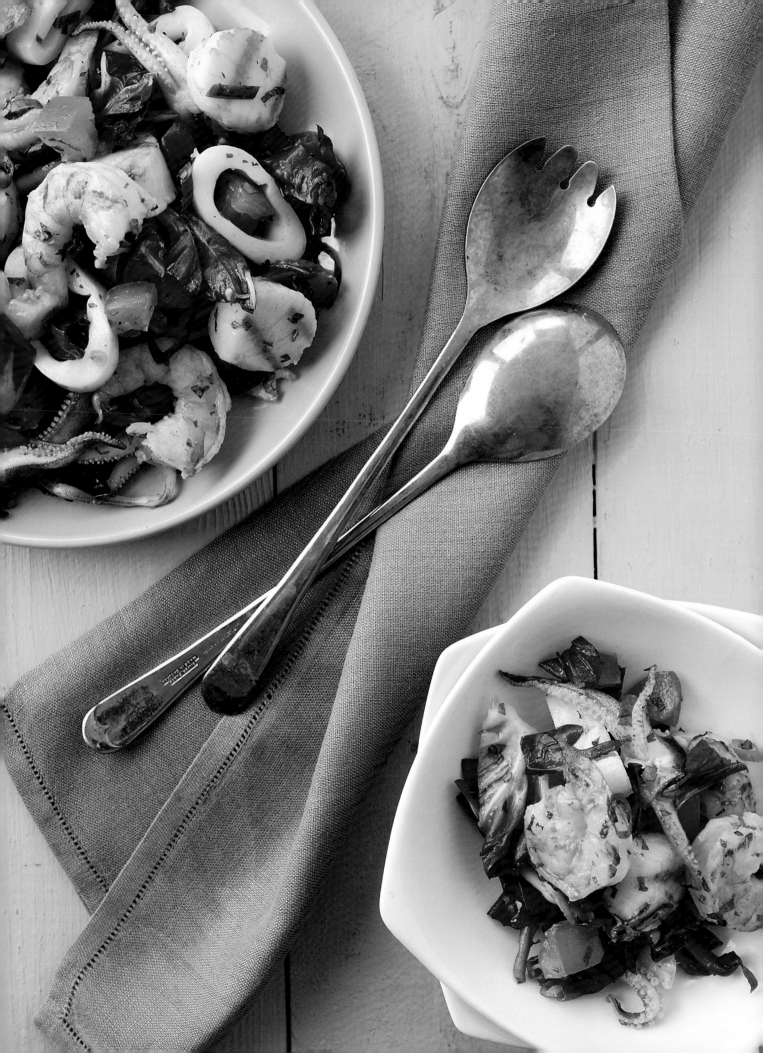

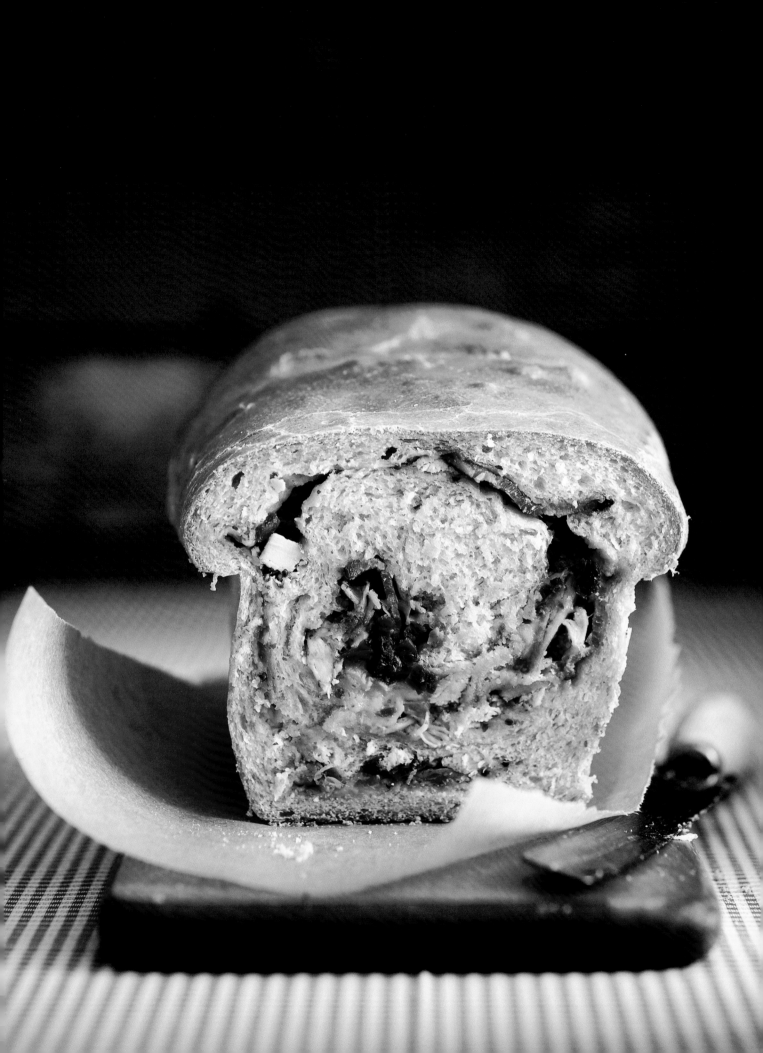

CLUB SANDWICH ROLL

Makes one 9- × 5-inch (23 × 12 cm) loaf • Serves 6 to 8

Talk about a portable sandwich. All the fillings you enjoy in a club sandwich are rolled into a soft, easy-to-make loaf of bread.

FRESH TAKE

- Adding olive oil to this bread dough makes it easy to work with, and keeps the baked loaf nice and soft, even if you chill the whole thing. (Typically bread dries out quickly in the fridge.)

- I found that, to make this recipe work, I had to use sun-dried tomatoes instead of fresh tomatoes, which you would expect on a club sandwich. Sun-dried to-matoes offer a concentrated tomato flavor without the sogginess of ripe tomatoes sitting on a sandwich for more than an hour.

- While we might associate a club sandwich with a good diner lunch or late-night hotel room service, my rec-ipe is intended for a picnic or to pack in a lunch, as it is mayonnaise-free, unlike the original.

Dough

2 cups	tepid water (105°F/41°C)	500 mL
2 Tbsp	cornmeal	30 mL
1 Tbsp	instant dry yeast	15 mL
1 Tbsp	honey or sugar	15 mL
3½–4 cups	all-purpose flour	875 mL–1 L
⅓ cup	olive oil	80 mL
2 tsp	salt	10 mL

Filling

8 strips	bacon, cooked	8 strips
3 cups	shredded honey mustard glazed chicken (page 65)	750 mL
2 cups	grated cheddar cheese	500 mL
⅓ cup	chopped sun-dried tomatoes	80 mL

For the dough, mix together the water, cornmeal, yeast, and honey or sugar and let sit for 5 minutes. Stir in 3½ cups (875 mL) flour, the olive oil, and salt and mix on low speed (if using a stand-up mixer with a dough hook) or stir by hand until the dough comes together. Add the remaining ½ cup (125 mL) flour if the dough is sticky and clings to the side of the bowl. Continue kneading on low speed with the mixer or turn the dough out and knead it by hand on a lightly floured surface until it feels elastic, about 5 minutes. Place the dough in a lightly oiled bowl, cover, and let sit in a draft-free place for 1 hour.

Once the dough has rested and doubled in size, turn it out onto a lightly floured surface and roll it out into a large 18- × 9-inch (45 × 23 cm) rectangle, just over ½ inch (1 cm) thick, with the shorter end facing you. Arrange the bacon slices lengthwise across the dough, sprinkle them with the shred-ded chicken, and top with the grated cheese and sun-dried tomatoes. Roll up the dough by the short end and place it in a greased 9- × 5-inch (23 × 12 cm) loaf pan. Cover the dough with a tea towel and let rest for 30 minutes.

Continued . . .

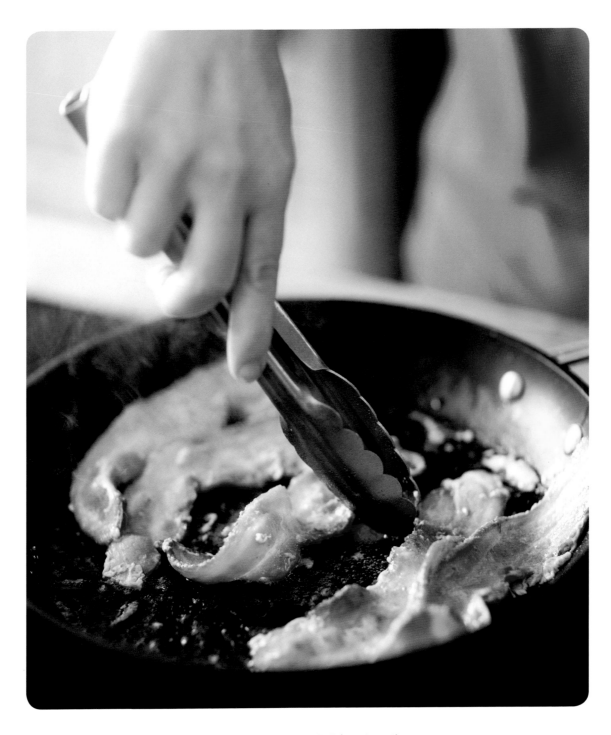

Club Sandwich Roll (continued)

Preheat the oven to 375°F (190°C).

Bake the sandwich roll for 20 minutes at 375°F (190°C). Reduce the oven temperature to 350°F (180°C) and bake for another 25 minutes. Let the roll cool for 15 minutes, then turn it out of the pan to cool for 30 minutes.

Slice and serve immediately, or chill it to serve cold.

GRILLED HALIBUT with TOMATO VINAIGRETTE

Serves 6

If you need something a bit dressier than an everyday tomato salsa, this dish is for you. The delicate texture of the flaky halibut is matched with a more refined tomato companion.

FRESH TAKE

- A professional in the kitchen makes use of every scrap of food, even what might seem to be waste. The tomato skins and seeds are packed with flavor, and letting them sit in the vinegar draws out every last bit of summery ripeness.

- Often halibut is sold in "steak" form, with bones in. You may have to order a few days ahead, but you can usually ask for fillet portions from the fish section at a good grocery store.

- Smoking meats on the grill by adding wood chips is common, but herbs can offer the same function. A trimming of thyme from your garden (even the tougher, woodier sprigs) creates a quick burst of herbaceous smoke that subtly contributes to a delicate fish. Be careful if you try this with rosemary, though—on the grill it can smell like the inside of a V W bus in 1967.

Tomato Vinaigrette

2	ripe beefsteak tomatoes	2
¼ cup	tomato vinegar (found at specialty food stores) or good-quality white wine vinegar	60 mL
1 tsp	minced garlic	5 mL
2 Tbsp	minced red onion	30 mL
¼ cup	good-quality extra virgin olive oil	60 mL
	salt & pepper	

Halibut

6	5 oz (150 g) halibut fillet portions	6
	olive oil, for brushing	
	salt & pepper	
1 bunch	fresh thyme sprigs	1 bunch
½ cup	loosely packed fresh basil leaves	125 mL

Mark the tomatoes with an X at the bottom and blanch for 1 minute in boiling water. Shock them in ice water then peel off the skins, reserving them for the vinaigrette. Remove and reserve the seeds and finely dice the tomato flesh.

Stir the vinegar and garlic with half the diced tomato and the reserved skins and seeds. Let sit for 30 minutes then strain it through a cheesecloth-lined strainer without squeezing (to keep the liquid clear). Dispose of the strained tomatoes, skins, and seeds (or add them to your next batch of chicken or vegetable stock). Whisk the red onion into the vinegar and slowly drizzle in the oil. Stir in the remaining half of the diced tomato and season to taste. Whisk the vinaigrette before using.

Preheat the grill on medium-high and heat a fish grill (mesh).

Brush the halibut fillets with oil and season lightly. Place the thyme on the grill. When it starts smoking, place the halibut fillets on the grill near but not on the thyme. Immediately close the lid on the barbecue and let the halibut cook for 8 minutes. Lift the lid, turn the halibut 90 degrees, and close the lid again. Cook the fish for 8 minutes more, until it flakes easily when touched with a fork. Remove the halibut from the grill and serve with the tomato vinaigrette. Tear basil leaves overtop immediately before serving.

Fish

POACHED SALMON with BASIL MOUSSELINE

Serves 8

Salmon is the best fish for poaching. It holds its shape and stays nice and moist, and its color sets beautifully once chilled. The mousseline sauce is mayonnaise-based with whipped cream folded in to make it fluffy. Rich, yes, but a little spoonful goes a long way.

FRESH TAKE

· Poaching is one of the leanest cooking methods you can use. I like to poach in the oven because it's easiest to maintain an even temperature. When poaching on the stove, you have to watch carefully that the liquid doesn't boil, as this would break apart the fish. By flavoring the poaching liquid in this recipe with lemon and herbs, you introduce complexity with subtlety.

· Poaching and chilling fish is also convenient if you're preparing ahead for a party, or if you want to cook early in the morning before the day gets too hot.

· The basil mousseline has other tasty uses. It's lovely spooned over chilled asparagus or green beans, or you can use it as an easy alternative to hollandaise on eggs Benedict.

Basil Mousseline

⅓ cup	mayonnaise	80 mL
½ cup	chopped fresh basil	125 mL
¼ cup	finely chopped green onion	60 mL
⅔ cup	whipping cream	160 mL
1 Tbsp	lemon juice	15 mL
	salt & pepper	

Poached Salmon

2 cups	dry white wine	500 mL
2 cups	water	500 mL
2	lemons, sliced	2
1	medium onion, sliced	1
2 sprigs	fresh oregano or dill	2 sprigs
8	5 oz (150 g) salmon fillet portions, skin-on and pin bones removed	8
	salt & pepper	
½ cup	finely diced red bell pepper, for garnish (optional)	125 mL

For the basil mousseline, add the mayonnaise, basil, and green onion to a food processor, pulse until blended, and scrape into a bowl. In another bowl, whip the cream to soft peaks and stir in the lemon juice. Fold the cream gently into the mayonnaise and season to taste. Chill for up to 6 hours.

Preheat the oven to 275°F (140°C). In a roasting pan or ovenproof *sauteuse* (sauté pan with tall sides), bring the wine, water, lemons, onion, and oregano or dill up to a simmer. Turn off the heat and add the salmon portions. Cover and transfer to the oven. Cook for 15 to 20 minutes, checking for doneness at 15 minutes. The salmon should have an internal temperature of 145°F (63°C) and the flesh should feel firm when gently pressed. Gently remove the salmon from the liquid using a slotted spoon, place it on a plate, and season lightly. Cool to room temperature then chill completely.

To serve, peel away the skin of the salmon and place the salmon on a plate or platter. Top with mousseline and sprinkle with red pepper, if desired. Serve cold.

Fish

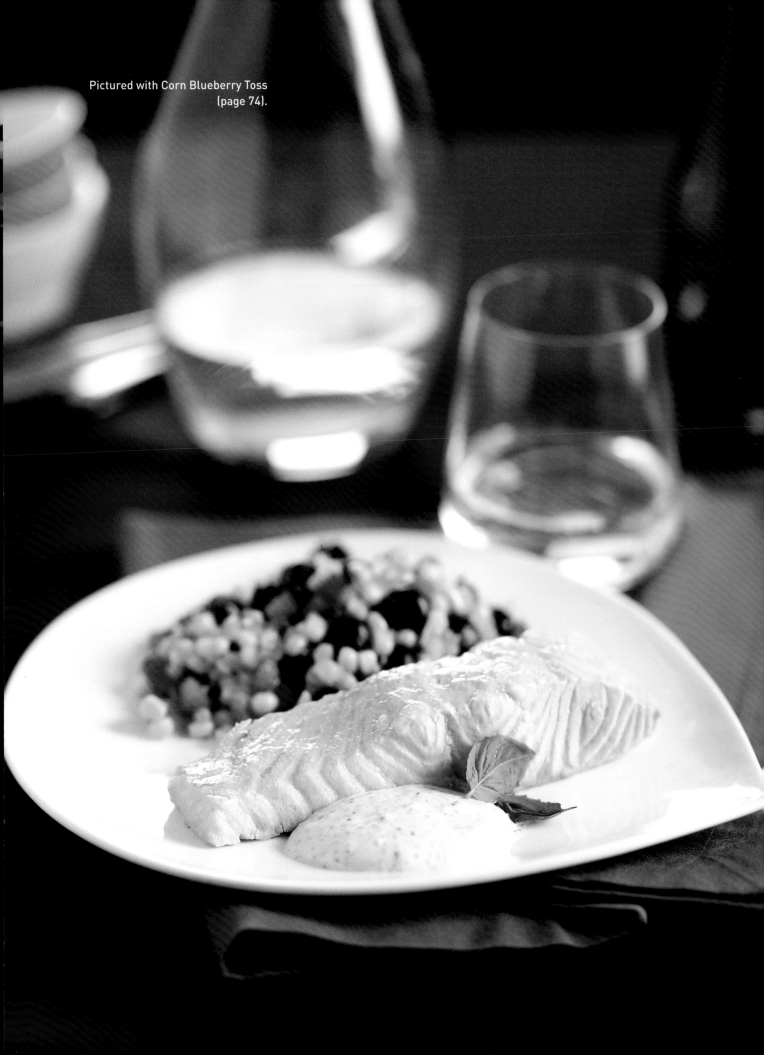

Pictured with Corn Blueberry Toss
(page 74).

HERB & VEGETABLE STUFFED STRIPED BASS

Serves 6

Striped bass has a mild taste and a lean texture, and served stuffed it is an appropriate size for one person. The presentation is fabulous if you are dining alfresco.

FRESH TAKE

- Small whole trout also suit this technique. If whole, dressed trout aren't available, you could even take two fillets and tie them together (a good option if you prefer not to stare at the head and tail on your plate).

- The choice of vegetables for stuffing the fish is based equally on their taste and their aromatic quality. As the fish cooks, the vegetables and herbs steam, emitting a fragrance that permeates every bite of the fish.

- To julienne is to cut into long thin strips. I chose this format not only for esthetics, but because it allows the vegetables to cook perfectly in time with the fish.

2	medium leeks, white and light green parts only	2
1	medium zucchini	1
1 stalk	celery	1 stalk
1	red bell pepper	1
3 Tbsp	white wine	45 mL
3 Tbsp	extra virgin olive oil	45 mL
	salt & pepper	
6	whole, cleaned striped bass (about 12 oz/ 375 g each), or other small whole fish	6
1	lemon, sliced thinly	1
12 sprigs	fresh thyme	12 sprigs
12	fresh basil leaves	12
	butcher's twine	

Julienne (cut into thin strips) the leeks, zucchini, celery, and red pepper. Toss them with the wine and olive oil and season lightly.

Preheat the grill to medium-high and place on a fish rack to heat (or make sure the grill is very clean). Rinse the striped bass, and fill the cavities with the julienne vegetables. Place a few lemon slices, 2 sprigs of thyme, and 2 basil leaves inside each fish. Using kitchen twine, tie each fish at the center (or in 2 places if necessary) to keep the vegetables in. Brush the outside of the fish with any remaining oil/wine from the bowl and season lightly. Place the fish on the heated grill rack and grill, without moving and with the barbecue uncovered, for about 8 minutes. Turn the fish over and cook, without moving again, for another 8 minutes, or until cooked through. Remove the twine and serve.

HONEY MUSTARD GLAZED CHICKEN

Makes 1 whole chicken • Serves 4 to 6

I like to serve this chicken right out of the oven, hot and sliced, but with chilled leftovers you really notice how great the glaze is. It sticks to the chicken, making the chicken taste fantastic on a sandwich or baked in the Club Sandwich Roll (page 59).

1	3½ lb (1.6 kg) chicken	1
1	onion, peeled and sliced, for roasting	1
2 Tbsp	olive oil	30 mL
	salt & pepper	
3	fresh thyme sprigs	3
½ cup	honey	125 mL
½ cup	coarse grain mustard	125 mL
1	small onion, for the glaze	1

Preheat the oven to 325°F (160°C).

Place the chicken on top of the sliced onion in a heavy-bottomed roasting pan and drizzle with oil. Season the chicken, insert the thyme sprigs into the cavity, cover, and roast for 20 minutes. Uncover and continue roasting until the internal temperature (taken between the thigh and breast) reads 180°F (82°C), about 1½ hours.

While the chicken is roasting, prepare the glaze. Whisk together the honey and mustard. Purée the onion as smoothly as possible and stir it into the honey mustard. During the last 45 minutes of cooking baste the chicken every 10 to 15 minutes with the honey mustard glaze. (Or you may wish to simply toss the cooked, cut-up chicken with the mixture.)

Poultry

Pictured with Tender Green Salad with Grilled Apricots & Red Onion Vinaigrette (page 47).

MARINATED FLANK STEAK *Serves 6 to 8*

Flank steak is the exception to the rule when it comes to grilled steaks. Typically we favor tender beef cuts like ribeye, New York striploin, and tenderloin, but flank steak, a tougher cut, really is tender when served sliced across the grain.

FRESH TAKE

- Flank steak is a tougher, leaner cut than even a sirloin. Marinating helps tenderize it, but the keys to success lie in grilling it no further than medium doneness to keep it moist, and slicing it on the bias so the knife cuts against the grain to create tender bitefuls.

- I like to serve most grilled items with a sprinkling of salt and pepper once they're on the plate. Slicing the meat exposes the center that doesn't get fully seasoned. The soy sauce marinade seasons this steak, but it may still need a little more salt to even out the balance.

- Why choose a flank steak over a more tender cut? While the more affordable cost is certainly a consideration, my real motivation is that flank steak has a full-bodied beef taste. Even a little taste is very fulfilling.

1 cup	red wine vinegar	250 mL
¼ cup	soy sauce	60 mL
2 Tbsp	Dijon mustard	30 mL
6 cloves	garlic, sliced	6 cloves
1	onion, sliced	1
3 sprigs	fresh rosemary	3 sprigs
2 Tbsp	olive oil	30 mL
2 lb	beef flank steak	1 kg
	coarse salt & cracked black pepper	

Stir together the vinegar, soy sauce, and mustard in a large flat dish. Stir in the garlic and onion. Pull the rosemary leaves off their stem and add. Whisk in the oil. Add the flank steak and spoon some of the marinade overtop the steak, along with the onion, garlic, and rosemary. Cover the dish and chill for at least 30 minutes and up to 12 hours before grilling, turning the steak once or twice.

To cook, preheat the grill to high. Grill the steak about 5 minutes on each side with the barbecue uncovered. Do not cook past medium doneness. Let the steak rest on a cutting board for 3 minutes before slicing on the bias (against the grain).

Arrange the steak on a salad (such as the one on page 47) or serving plate and season with salt and pepper before serving.

Meat

DRY-GLAZED PORK TENDERLOIN *Serves 6*

What begins as a rub, adding complexity to an easy-to-grill pork tenderloin, melts into a gooey glaze, caramelizing onto the pork by the time it has finished cooking.

FRESH TAKE

- You don't want to press the rub onto the tenderloin more than an hour before grilling. If the rub sits too long on the pork in the fridge it will start melting and then become a glaze before you want it to.

- The cream of tartar adds a dry form of acidity to the rub so that you're not adding liquid in the form of vinegar or lemon juice, which would dissolve the rub. That little hit of acidity heightens the flavor. (Cream of tartar is normally an ingredient in marinades and barbecue sauces.)

- Serve this pork tenderloin with any of your favorite summertime side dishes—potato salad, grilled vegetables, or even just sliced ripe tomatoes.

Dry Glaze

⅔ cup	packed light brown sugar	160 mL
3 cloves	garlic, minced	3 cloves
1 Tbsp	finely grated orange zest	15 mL
3 Tbsp	paprika	45 mL
1 Tbsp	sesame seeds	15 mL
1 Tbsp	ground ginger	15 mL
1 Tbsp	ground coriander	15 mL
2 tsp	fine sea salt	10 mL
2 tsp	ground black pepper	10 mL
1 tsp	cream of tartar	5 mL

Pork

3	pork tenderloins (about 1 lb/500 g each)	3

For the dry glaze, stir together the brown sugar, garlic, and orange zest to blend. In a separate bowl, stir together the remaining ingredients and add them to the brown sugar mixture. Set the glaze aside until ready to use.

Clean the pork tenderloin of any connective tissue.

Preheat the grill to medium and clean it well.

Rub the tenderloins completely with the dry glaze and immediately place on the grill. Grill, uncovered, for about 8 minutes on each side, rotating 90 degrees halfway through grilling each side, until an internal temperature of 155°F (68°C) is reached. Let the pork sit for a moment before slicing and serving.

GARLIC COLESLAW *Makes about 6 cups (1.5 l)*

This simple coleslaw is a universal favorite with guests and with staff at the bakery. It's no wonder I end up making it at home for Michael and me so often.

FRESH TAKE

· Any variety of green cabbage is tasty in this recipe. I often like to use Savoy cabbage for its unique character—it has light green leaves on the outside, yielding to tender and mild yellow leaves on the inside. But when local green-head cabbage is in season, I can't resist. One head of cabbage can feed 20 people!

· There's something inherently simple and comforting about this coleslaw. Maybe it's the sweet intensity of the maple syrup and raisins against the raw garlic. Whatever it is, it's summertime comfort food.

· If the oomph of raw garlic is a little too much for you or your crowd, try blanching the garlic first. Covering garlic cloves with boiling water and letting it cool takes the edge off the garlic but still keeps it tasting fresh.

Dressing		
¼ cup	mayonnaise	60 mL
¼ cup	sour cream	60 mL
2 Tbsp	lemon juice	30 mL
2 Tbsp	pure maple syrup	30 mL
2 cloves	garlic, minced	2 cloves
	salt & pepper	

Slaw		
6 cups	finely sliced green cabbage	1.5 L
3	green onions, sliced on a bias	3
⅔ cup	golden raisins	160 mL
½ cup	lightly toasted walnut pieces	125 mL

Whisk all the dressing ingredients and season lightly.

Toss the cabbage, green onions, raisins, and walnuts with the dressing and adjust seasoning.

Vegetables

CORN BLUEBERRY TOSS *Serves 6*

This vegetable side dish is all about those vibrant colors of summer. Served alongside grilled fish, chicken, or even steak, its bright color is matched only by its palate-awakening combination of fruit, vegetable, and a little heat. (Pictured on page 63.)

(Pictured on page 63.)

FRESH TAKE

- My friend Maggie Babcock inspired this recipe. Years ago I attended a garden party at her home. While I had often hosted cooking class dinners in her home in years prior, this time the host was teaching me a thing or two—this toss is a prime example.

- Fresh blueberries have a white film over them that, even when washed, stays on them (as it's supposed to). But when the blueberries are tossed with lime juice and a little bit of olive oil, the "blue" in the blueberry jumps to life and contrasts beautifully with the red bell pepper, green onion, and yellow corn.

- The candied ginger is my little secret addition—little bites of unexpected sweet heat. Try adding a little diced candied ginger to a bowl of fresh summer berries for a pleasant surprise.

4 ears	fresh corn (about 3 cups/750 mL kernels)	4 ears
2 Tbsp	extra virgin olive oil	30 mL
⅔ cup	chopped green onion	160 mL
1	red bell pepper, finely diced	1
1½ cups	fresh blueberries	375 mL
2 Tbsp	lime juice	30 mL
1 Tbsp	chopped fresh cilantro	15 mL
1	jalapeño pepper, seeded and finely chopped (optional)	1
1 Tbsp	finely chopped candied ginger	15 mL
	salt & pepper	

Remove corn kernels from ears. In a medium sauté pan over medium heat, add the oil and then the corn. Sauté until the corn is tender and bright, about 3 minutes, and remove to cool. In a large bowl toss the remaining ingredients with the corn and season to taste.

This salad can be prepared up to a day ahead and chilled until ready to serve.

Vegetables

HERB GRILLED CORN-ON-THE-COB *Serves 6*

When corn is in season, enjoying it right on the cob is the ideal way to appreciate it—in its original serving format. But while I appreciate the classic butter and salt combination, sometimes I look for that little something extra, especially if I'm entertaining.

FRESH TAKE

- The butter recipe I make here is known as a compound butter. Dollop the same concoction on a grilled steak or a baked potato, or use it to baste a grilled or roasted chicken breast.

- Corn silk is one of my pet peeves, because if it's not properly cleaned off the ears of corn it interferes with every bite. Yes, I need dental floss after eating corn-on-the-cob, not during!

- Adding grated Parmesan right before serving is inspired by the Mexican street food treat of corn-on-the-cob slathered in mayo then sprinkled with grated Mexican cheese.

½ cup	unsalted butter, at room temperature	125 mL
½ cup	chopped green onion	125 mL
3 Tbsp	chopped fresh oregano	45 mL
3 Tbsp	chopped fresh cilantro	45 mL
6 ears	corn-on-the-cob, with husks on	6 ears
¾ cup	finely grated Parmesan	185 mL

In a food processor, pulse the butter with the green onion, oregano, and cilantro until smooth.

Gently peel back the husk of the corn and pull off the silk. Rub each ear generously with the herb butter. Fold back the husks to cover the corn, tie the tops of the husks with twine, and chill for at least 20 minutes and up to a day.

Preheat the grill to medium-high.

Grill the corn for about 18 minutes, turning it occasionally to cook evenly. Serve the corn in its husk and allow your guests to peel the corn and sprinkle it with grated Parmesan to their liking.

Vegetables

HEIRLOOM TOMATO SALAD *Serves 6*

The stunning array of colors of heirloom tomatoes is just the beginning of the simple perfection of this salad. The sweetness, tartness, and texture of each tomato vary as much as the size and color.

FRESH TAKE

• Heirloom tomatoes should be appreciated in their most basic state. Even a vinaigrette will blur the varied and unique tastes of a selection of tomato varieties served together. A little olive oil, salt, and pepper are all that is needed to heighten the flavors that are already there.

• True heirloom tomatoes are open-pollinated, meaning they are not hybrid, although how far back the origins of the seeds can be traced is a topic of debate. There are heirloom tomato co-operatives, and as a purchasing farmer, you must agree to save and send back to the co-op the same number of seeds you purchased to replenish the stock.

• Heirloom tomatoes can have some great names: Bull's Blood, Mars Stripe, Brandy-wine, Cherokee Purple—they taste as fanciful as they sound.

2 lb	a variety of heirloom or peak-season tomatoes	1 kg
	good-quality extra virgin olive oil	
	fine quality sea salt	
	ground black pepper	

Slice the tomatoes and arrange them on a platter. Drizzle them with olive oil, and season with salt and pepper. Serve at room temperature.

Vegetables

SUMMER SUNSHINE SMOOTHIES *Serves 4*

Like a ray of sunshine, this thick, creamy concoction is the best way to start your day. Truly, breakfast in a glass.

FRESH TAKE

- For a kick of fiber, I also like to stir in a spoonful of toasted wheat germ. It softens up in the smoothie, and adds a subtle and pleasant nuttiness.

- I find that sometimes I don't even need the honey because the sweetness of the fruit is enough to balance the tart yogurt. Give the smoothie a taste first, and then decide if you need the honey.

- If you freeze summertime fruits, this smoothie in the midst of winter truly does earn its "sunshine" title.

2 cups	peeled and diced peaches	500 mL
1 cup	diced fresh apricots	250 mL
1 cup	diced banana	250 mL
2 cups	yogurt (low-fat is fine)	500 mL
½ cup	milk (low-fat is fine)	125 mL
1 tsp	vanilla extract	5 mL
1 Tbsp	chopped fresh mint	15 mL
3 Tbsp	honey	45 mL
2–3 cups	ice cubes	500–750 mL
	fresh mint sprigs, for garnish	

Add all the ingredients except the ice to a blender and purée until smooth. Add the ice and pulse to crush. Pour the mixture into 4 tall glasses, garnish with mint sprigs, and serve immediately.

Alternatively, the mixture can be blended (without the ice) up to 3 hours in advance and poured over ice to serve.

Breakfast

FRUIT ANTIPASTI *Serves 6*

Need something other than a fruit cup? This arrangement of fruits offers simplicity and sophistication all in one go.

FRESH TAKE

- I have always loved how sweet, low-acidity fruits like melon can be brought to life with a little lime juice. Sprinkled with colorful blueberries, this dish goes from boringly basic to stunningly spectacular.

- Rooibos tea is a fluoride-laden, caffeine-free flavor burst that is perfect as an infusion for citrus. Think outside the box (or the bag, as it were). Tea is a great flavor enhancer, and can be used to flavor anything from custards to barbecue sauce, in almost any recipe where liquid is gently heated and tea can be infused.

- Yum! Peaches and blackberries are at their peak together, so they're meant to be enjoyed together. A breakfast-y hint of maple and cinnamon sparkles them up for a sunrise.

HONEYDEW BLUEBERRY WITH LIME

1 Tbsp	honey	15 mL
1 tsp	finely grated lime zest	5 mL
1 Tbsp	lime juice	15 mL
½	honeydew melon, peeled and seeded	½
1 cup	fresh blueberries	250 mL

Stir the honey and lime zest and juice to blend. Slice the honeydew as thinly as possible. Arrange the melon and berries in a bowl or on a platter and spoon the honey mixture overtop.

GRAPEFRUIT WATERMELON WITH ROOIBOS TEA

2	red grapefruit	2
1	rooibos tea bag	1
2 Tbsp	honey	30 mL
2 cups	diced watermelon, cut into 1-inch (2.5 cm) pieces	500 mL

Peel the grapefruit, including the membrane, using a serrated knife. Cut away the grapefruit segments from the membrane over a bowl to reserve the juices. Heat the juices with the rooibos tea and honey over low heat until warm. Let the tea bag sit for 10 minutes then remove and let the tea cool. Gently toss the grapefruit and watermelon with the tea mixture and chill until ready to serve.

PEACH BLACKBERRY WITH CINNAMON MAPLE

¼ cup	pure maple syrup	60 mL
½ tsp	ground cinnamon	2 mL
3 cups	peeled and sliced peaches	750 mL
1 cup	fresh blackberries	250 mL

Stir the maple syrup and cinnamon to combine. Toss in the peaches and blackberries and chill until ready to serve.

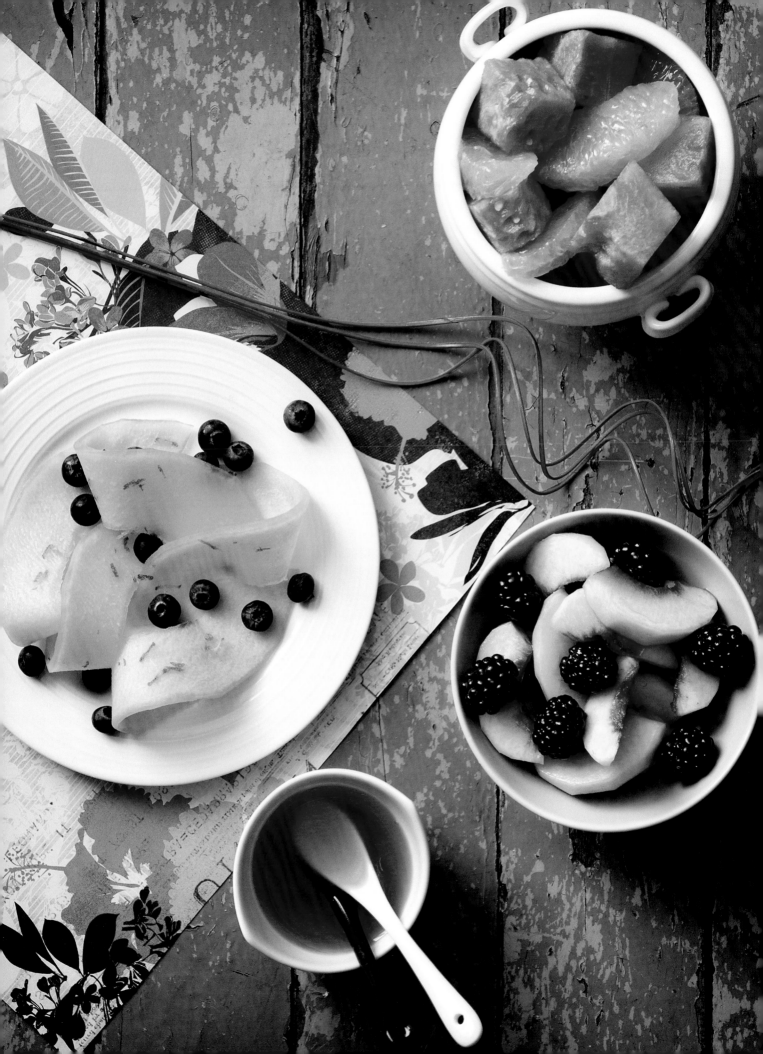

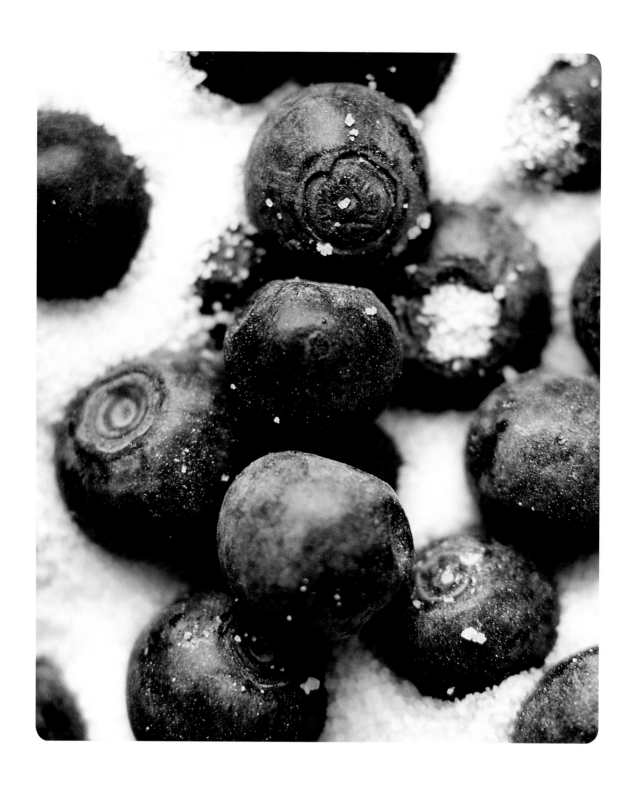

BLUEBERRY STICKY BUNS *Makes 12 sticky buns*

Love a good cinnamon bun? Love a blueberry muffin fresh out of the oven? Well, meet your next true love—these sticky buns are a perfect marriage of these two breakfast treats.

FRESH TAKE

- That little bit of nutmeg is my secret to a great sticky-bun dough—it adds that familiar "donut" element that takes these to the next level.

- To make these for breakfast or brunch without waking at five a.m., make the dough and assemble the sticky buns, filled and in the pan, and pop the pan in the fridge the night before. In the morning, pull them out while you preheat the oven and get the coffee going, and before you know it, the buns are baking.

- Don't limit the fruit filling to mere blueberries. Raspberries, sliced peaches, apples, or even fresh or frozen cranberries make these sticky buns seasonal and delectable.

Dough

2 tsp	instant dry yeast	10 mL
1	egg, at room temperature	1
½ cup	milk, at room temperature	125 mL
2 Tbsp	sugar	30 mL
2½ cups	all-purpose flour	625 mL
½ tsp	salt	2 mL
½ tsp	ground nutmeg	2 mL
½ cup	unsalted butter, at room temperature	125 mL
½ cup	cream cheese, at room temperature	125 mL

Sticky Bun Filling

1 cup	packed brown sugar	250 mL
½ cup	unsalted butter, at room temperature	125 mL
3 Tbsp	pure maple syrup	45 mL
1 Tbsp	ground cinnamon	15 mL
2 cups	fresh or frozen blueberries	500 mL

For the dough, dissolve the yeast in ¼ cup (60 mL) warm water in the bowl of a stand mixer fitted with a dough hook (or with electric beaters fitted with dough hooks) and allow to sit for 5 minutes.

Add the egg, milk, and sugar and blend. Add the flour, salt, and nutmeg and mix for 1 minute to combine. Add the butter and cream cheese and knead for 5 minutes on medium speed. Place the dough in a lightly oiled bowl, cover, and let rest for 1 hour.

Grease the cups of a 12-cup muffin tin.

For the filling, combine the sugar, butter, maple syrup, and cinnamon. Spoon a tablespoonful (15 mL) of filling into the bottom of each cup of the prepared muffin tin.

On a lightly floured surface, roll out the dough into a rectangle ½ inch (1 cm) thick. Spread the remaining filling over the dough, sprinkle with blueberries, and roll the dough up lengthwise. Slice it into 12 equal portions and arrange 1 portion in each muffin cup. Allow the dough to rise for half an hour loosely covered by a clean tea towel.

Preheat the oven to 350°F (180°C).

Bake the buns for 30 minutes, and turn out onto a plate while still warm.

This is a fruit-laden coffee cake that slices easily. The fruits can be anything in season, from rhubarb through to apples, but midsummer's apricots and plums are my preference.

FRESH TAKE

- *Platz* is simply German for square. This coffee cake is sometimes sold at fruit stalls at the farmers' markets that I go to. You can buy a basket of plums, and at the same time a square of coffee cake baked with those same plums. It's a local treat.

- If you opt for baking this *platz* with a mix of berries it has an elegant taste and texture, and suits a scoop of ice cream at the end of a summer supper.

1 cup	sugar	250 mL
¾ cup	unsalted butter, at room temperature	185 mL
¼ cup	full-fat sour cream	60 mL
4	large eggs, at room temperature	4
1 tsp	vanilla extract	5 mL
½ tsp	almond extract	2 mL
1 cup	all-purpose flour	250 mL
⅓ cup	ground almonds	80 mL
2 tsp	finely grated lemon zest	10 mL
1½ tsp	baking powder	7.5 mL
¼ tsp	ground nutmeg	1 mL
¼ tsp	salt	1 mL
2 cups	mixed fresh fruit, such as apricot halves, peach slices, plum halves and/ or mixed berries	500 mL
	sugar and ground cinnamon, for sprinkling	

Preheat the oven to 350°F (180°C). Grease a 9- × 13-inch (23 × 33 cm) pan.

Beat the sugar and butter until light and fluffy. Beat in the sour cream, then add the eggs one at a time, beating well after each addition. Stir in the vanilla and almond extracts. In a separate bowl, stir the flour, ground almonds, lemon zest, baking powder, nutmeg, and salt to combine. Add this to the butter mixture and stir just until incorporated. Spread the batter into the prepared pan and arrange the fruit overtop, pressing it in gently. If you're using plums or apricots halves, arrange them with their flat side up. Sprinkle lightly with sugar and cinnamon and bake for 25 to 30 minutes, until a tester inserted in the center of the cake comes out clean.

Cool completely before slicing into squares and serving.

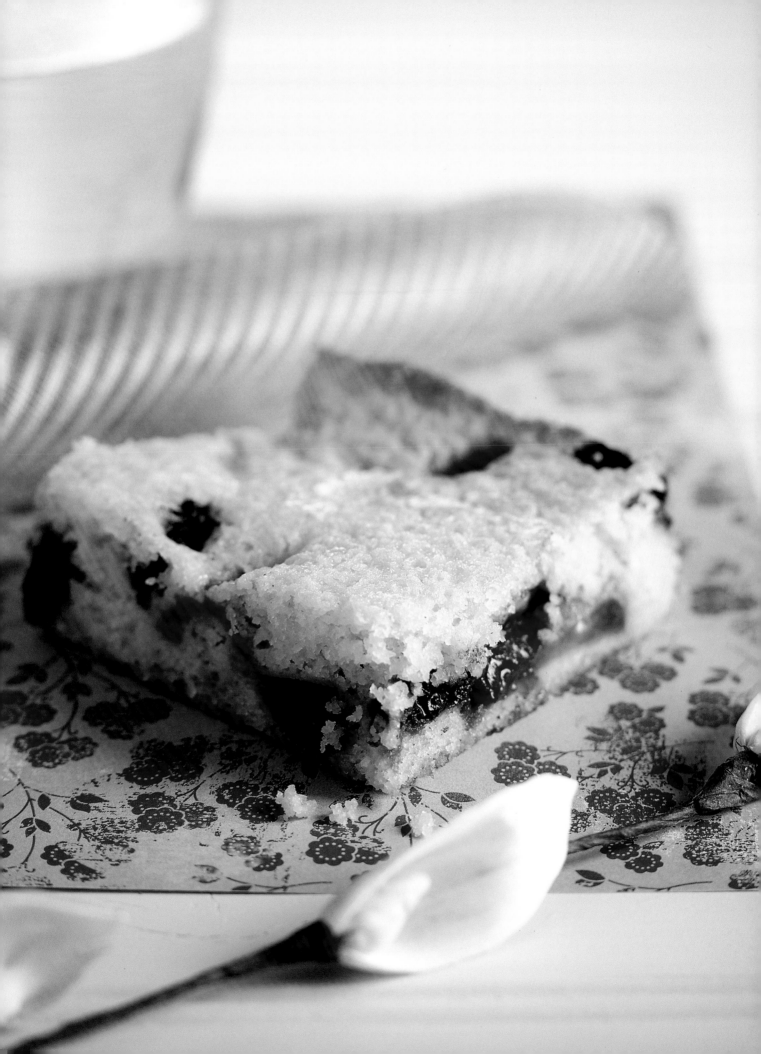

SUMMER FRUITS with ICEWINE SABAYON

Serves 8

Sabayon could be described as a meringue of egg yolks—it's frothy and light just like a meringue, but has a custardlike richness of its own.

FRESH TAKE

- Like a liqueur, icewine is enjoyed in small portions, so I like to open a bottle when we're having a few couples over. The sabayon only takes a few tablespoons, so there'll still be enough for everyone.

- I enjoy sabayon served warm, as originally intended, but the way I serve it here—making it ahead and chilling it—is just as refreshing.

- Icewine is such a Canadian treat. Leave it to Canadians to serve and enjoy one of the best things winter has to offer in the middle of summer!

6	egg yolks	6
6 Tbsp	sugar	90 mL
3 Tbsp	lemon juice	45 mL
3 Tbsp	icewine or other sweet dessert wine, such Moscato	45 mL
2 Tbsp	whipping cream	30 mL
6 cups	fresh seasonal fruits (sliced peaches, berries, apricots, etc.)	1.5 L

Whisk the egg yolks, sugar, lemon juice, and icewine in a metal or glass bowl until combined. Place the bowl over a pot of gently simmering water (making sure that the bowl does not touch) and whisk constantly until the mixture doubles in volume and holds a "ribbon" when the whisk is lifted. Remove from the heat and stir in the cream. Chill until ready to serve.

To serve, arrange fresh fruits in parfait glasses or fruit cups. Spoon sabayon overtop the fruit.

The sabayon can be made and chilled up to a day in advance.

APRICOT PRESERVES *Makes about 6 cups (1.5 l)*

This is not your Tuesday morning jam to spread on toast. I find this has a little more elegance and certainly complexity, fit for high tea with scones, served alongside cheese, or as a filling for a tart.

FRESH TAKE

· The combination of lemon zest, ginger, and lavender gives this preserve its layers of flavor, which is why I like it particularly with cheese. I build a cheese platter with a creamy brie, a nutty washed-rind cheese, and a pungent blue. The apricot goes with all three styles of cheese.

· Apricots have to be the easiest fruit to prepare for preserving, second only to blueberries and raspberries. Just a wash, no peeling, and with apricots, a quick score around the fruit and a twist to pop out the pit.

· Fresh lavender tastes best when it's flowering, but you can use the lavender stems and leaves if the season for flowers has passed. I prefer to have the lavender wrapped in cheesecloth; if I don't do this, the buds fall off the stem and turn black, looking rather like insects swimming in the preserve.

· Following safe canning procedures is important if "putting up" preserves to store unrefrigerated over the winter. Visit a trust-worthy website like www .homecanning.ca (or ".com" in the U.S.) for details.

1 lb	pitted fresh apricots, cut into quarters	500 g
3 cups	sugar	750 mL
1 cup	honey	250 mL
3 Tbsp	finely grated lemon zest	45 mL
3 Tbsp	lemon juice	45 mL
2 Tbsp	freshly grated ginger	30 mL
6–8 stems	fresh lavender (flowering)	6–8 stems
1 pouch	(6 fl oz/175 mL) liquid pectin	1 pouch

Bring the apricots, sugar, honey, lemon zest and juice, and ginger to a simmer, stirring often. Wrap the lavender in a piece of cheesecloth and add it to the simmering fruit for about 8 minutes, until the apricots are tender. Remove the lavender and stir in the pectin.

Remove from the heat and jar according to proper canning procedures, or pack it in plastic or glass containers and refrigerate.

Opened preserves and preserves that don't go through the canning process will keep refrigerated for up to 4 months.

BABY CHERRY PIES *Makes 12 mini pies or one 9-inch (23 cm) pie*

These gems look just like the full-sized original. I've included instructions for the classic cherry pie here as well, in case that suits your occasion better.

FRESH TAKE

- Sweet cherries are more commonly found in the produce section of the grocery store and are meant for eating, whereas tart cherries are bright and tangy and perfect for jams and pies. It can be a challenge to find *fresh* tart cherries as their season is short. I buy mine pitted and frozen when the season's passed.

- For the baby pie lattice tops, I find it much easier to make a full-sized lattice and then cut out mini rounds with a cookie cutter. I couldn't imagine rolling, cutting, and weaving 12 separate lattice tops.

- I weave a lattice pattern by laying out half the pastry strips in a row, with just a ¼-inch (6 mm) gap in between each strip. Then I pull back every other strip halfway and lay another pastry strip across, right at the folds. I unfold the pastry and then fold every other strip the other way and lay another strip across. I repeat this process in both directions. Working from the middle of the lattice out means handling the pastry as little as possible and keeping it cool, which prevents cracking.

Crust

2½ cups	all-purpose flour	625 mL
½ tsp	fine sea salt	2 mL
½ cup	cold unsalted butter, cut into pieces	125 mL
½ cup	cold vegetable shortening, cut into pieces	125 mL
2 Tbsp	lemon juice	30 mL
4–8 Tbsp	cold water	60–125 mL

Cherry Filling

6 cups	pitted tart cherries, fresh or frozen	1.5 L
1½ cups	sugar	375 mL
pinch	ground cinnamon	pinch
¼ cup	cornstarch	60 mL
1	egg mixed with 2 Tbsp (30 mL) cold water, for brushing	1
	sugar and ground cinnamon, for sprinkling	

For the crust, combine the flour with the salt. Cut in the butter and shortening until the dough has a rough, crumbly texture. Add the lemon juice and 4 Tbsp (60 mL) of the water and blend just until the dough comes together, and if needed adding more water 1 Tbsp (15 mL) at a time to bring the dough together. Shape into a disk (2 disks if making 1 regular pie), wrap, and chill for 30 minutes.

For the filling, bring the cherries, sugar, and cinnamon up to a simmer. Cook for 15 minutes, stirring often. Whisk the cornstarch with ¼ cup (60 mL) cold water and stir it into the cherries. Cook until thickened, then remove from the heat and let cool.

Preheat the oven to 375°F (190°C).

For 12 mini pies, roll out two-thirds of the dough and cut out circles to line 12 regular muffin cups. Fill the cups with cherry filling. Roll out the remaining dough to a square and cut it into ½-inch (1 cm) strips. On a lightly floured surface, make a lattice-top pattern (see Fresh Take). Then,

Continued . . .

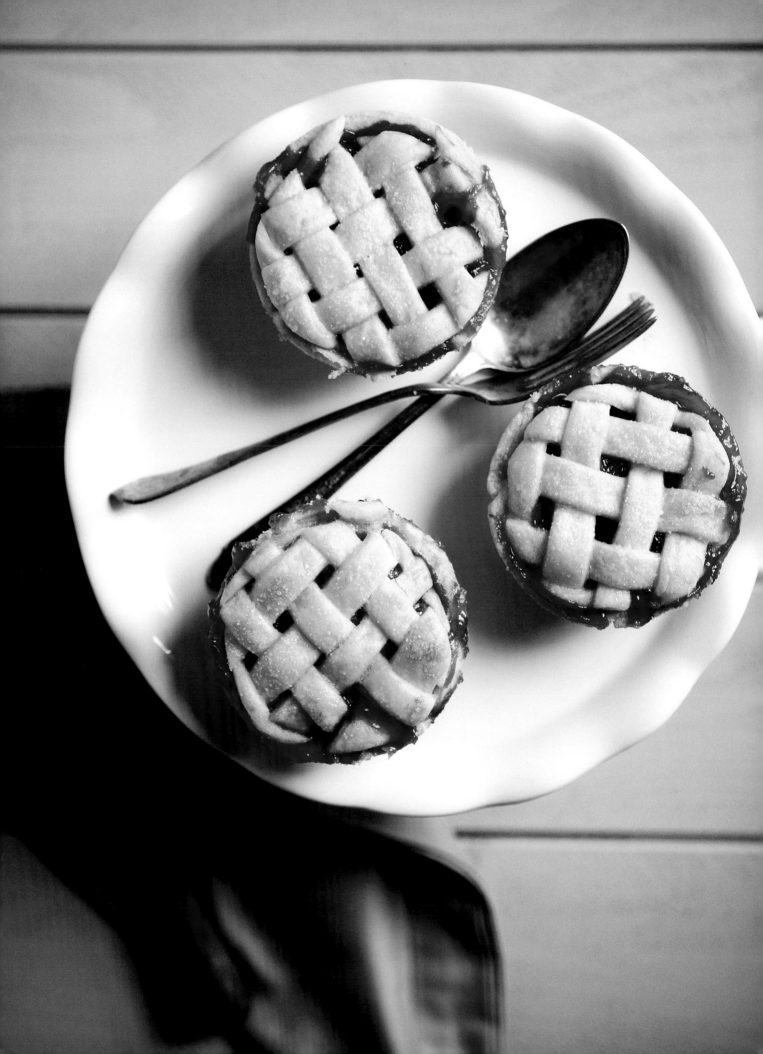

with a 2½-inch (6 cm) cookie cutter, cut out 12 lattice tops. Use a spatula to gently place a lattice top on each pie, cinching the edges gently. Brush with the egg wash, sprinkle with sugar and cinnamon, and bake for 5 minutes, then reduce the oven temperature to 350°F (180°C) and bake for about 25 minutes.

For a regular pie, preheat the oven to 400°F (200°C). On a lightly floured surface, roll out one of the disks into a circle large enough to fit a 9-inch (23 cm) pie pan. Line the pan with the pastry and trim the edges. Spoon cherry filling into the shell. Roll out the second piece of dough to fit on top and cut a 1-inch (2.5 cm) hole in its center. Brush the pie with the egg wash and sprinkle with sugar and cinnamon. Place the pie pan on a baking tray and bake for 15 minutes. Reduce the oven temperature to 375°F (190°C) and continue baking until the crust is a rich golden brown. Cool the pie for an hour before slicing.

PEACH FROZEN YOGURT *Makes about 6 cups (1.5 l)*

Hands down, peach frozen yogurt is my absolute favorite flavor in frozen yogurt, and this one is definitely peachy!

FRESH TAKE

- As you can see, this recipe has more peaches than anything else. It really has a sorbet character to it, and a lovely blush tone into the bargain.

- While this recipe is indeed quite lean, I find that the whipping cream is needed to keep the texture of the frozen yogurt smooth and not icy.

- Because the base for the frozen yogurt is not heated (like custard ice creams), using superfine (berry) sugar is recommended as it dissolves more easily into the peaches.

4 cups	peeled and diced fresh peaches	1 L
½ cup	superfine sugar (berry sugar)	125 mL
2 Tbsp	lemon juice	30 mL
1 tsp	vanilla extract	5 mL
2 cups	yogurt (low-fat is fine)	500 mL
¾ cup	whipping cream, whipped to soft peaks	185 mL

Purée the peaches in a blender until smooth. Blend in the sugar, lemon juice, and vanilla until the sugar has dissolved. Pulse in the yogurt until the mixture is smooth. Fold in the whipped cream and process in an ice cream maker, following the manufacturer's instructions. Scrape the frozen yogurt into a nonreactive container and freeze further until firm, at least 3 hours.

FRENCH CUSTARD ICE CREAM with WINE-STEEPED PLUMS *Serves 6*

A luscious homemade ice cream is only made better when served with luscious fruits. The wine-steeped plums are only barely softened by a warm wine mixture before they mix and meld with the ice cream as it slowly melts in the dish.

FRESH TAKE

· I find it worthwhile to whisk the eggs and sugar over a water bath to cook the eggs a little and to build air into the custard, making for an exceptionally smooth-textured ice cream.

· When I steep the plums this way, it's just to soften them a bit and impart flavor. Any longer at a simmer and I'd have to rename them stewed plums—not nearly as appealing.

· It would also be a lovely twist to steep the plums in a ruby port in place of the red wine. Serving the plums and ice cream with port is also highly recommended.

2 cups	whipping cream, divided	500 mL
½ cup	2% milk	125 mL
1	vanilla bean	1
4	egg yolks	4
⅓ cup	sugar	80 mL
pinch	salt	pinch
pinch	ground cinnamon	pinch

For the ice cream, heat 1 cup (250 mL) of the cream and the milk and scrape out the seeds of the vanilla bean (add the vanilla pod to steep in the cream for extra flavor). Keep to just below a simmer.

In a bowl over a pot of gently simmering water, whisk the egg yolks, sugar, salt, and cinnamon vigorously until thick and a pale buttery color, about 3 minutes. Remove the bowl from the heat. Remove the vanilla pod from the heated cream and slowly ladle the cream into the eggs, whisking constantly until all the cream has been added. Return the mixture to medium heat and stir with a wooden spoon until it coats the spoon, about 3 minutes. Strain through a fine-mesh sieve and chill the mixture completely.

Whip the remaining 1 cup (250 mL) cream to soft peaks and fold it into the chilled custard. Freeze in an ice cream maker, following the manufacturer's instructions, then scrape into a container and freeze until firm, about 2 hours.

WINE-STEEPED PLUMS

½ cup	sugar	125 mL
½ cup	dry red wine	125 mL
2	cinnamon sticks	2
¼ tsp	ground cloves	1 mL
6	large red plums (or 10 Italian prune plums)	6

In a pot, bring the sugar and wine up to a simmer with the cinnamon sticks and cloves, cooking until the sugar has dissolved. Pit the plums and cut them into quarters. Add the plums to the wine mixture and bring to a simmer. As soon as a simmer is reached, remove the pot from the heat and strain the liquid into a small pot. Reduce the liquid by half then return it to the plums.

Serve warm with the ice cream. If preparing these plums beforehand, store in the refrigerator.

CHOCOLATE GRIDDLE CAKES with
CINNAMON PEACHES *Makes 12 large (5-inch • 12 cm) pancakes*

While I think of these griddle cakes as dessert more than breakfast, they might be a fun way to start a special day. A birthday breakfast, perhaps?

FRESH TAKE

- These griddle cakes and peaches could also be a fabulous dessert served with a little ice cream, and maybe a drizzle of chocolate sauce.

- It doesn't matter here whether you use Dutch process or regular cocoa powder. It's more in baking that the difference in acidity matters (it's the acidity that differentiates the two types).

- Add slices of banana to the griddle cakes as you cook them, or replace the peaches with banana, for an altogether different treat.

1¼ cups	all-purpose flour	310 mL
¼ cup	cocoa powder	60 mL
3 Tbsp	sugar	45 mL
1½ tsp	baking powder	7.5 mL
½ tsp	baking soda	2 mL
¼ tsp	salt	1 mL
1⅔ cups	buttermilk, at room temperature	410 mL
3 Tbsp	unsalted butter, melted	45 mL
2	large eggs, at room temperature	2
1 tsp	vanilla extract	5 mL
1 cup	semisweet chocolate chips	250 mL
	oil, for greasing	

Sift the flour, cocoa, sugar, baking powder, baking soda, and salt. In a separate bowl, whisk together the buttermilk, melted butter, eggs, and vanilla. Add the buttermilk mixture to the flour mixture and stir just until combined (a few lumps are okay). Stir in the chocolate chips.

Preheat the oven to 200°F (95°C). Preheat a griddle over medium heat and grease with oil.

Ladle the batter onto the griddle to make 5-inch (12 cm) pancakes and cook for about 3 minutes. Turn once and cook for another 2 minutes. Transfer the griddle cakes to a plate, cover, and keep warm in the oven until ready to serve.

CINNAMON PEACHES
Makes about 2 cups (500 ml)

¼ cup	pure maple syrup	60 mL
2 Tbsp	unsalted butter	30 mL
6	peaches, peeled and sliced	6
½ tsp	ground cinnamon	2 mL

Bring the maple syrup and butter to a simmer in a large sauté pan. Stir in the peaches and cinnamon and return to a simmer. Serve immediately, spooned over the griddle cakes.

PLUM CLAFOUTIS *Serves 6*

Clafoutis is a simple and classic French bistro dessert and, like a crème brûlée, is meant to be served in the dish in which it's baked.

FRESH TAKE

- The batter for clafoutis is very much like a crêpe batter. Its function is to frame and hold the fruit in place. The original clafoutis uses whole sweet cherries (pits and all), but plums have a comparable color and texture (and definitely pits out).

- A drizzle of honey is an elegant way to finish this dessert. To make lavender honey, heat ½ cup (125 mL) honey with about six sprigs of fresh lavender over low heat for 15 minutes. Strain immediately and let cool before using.

4	purple plums or Italian prune plums	4
½ cup	all-purpose flour	125 mL
6 Tbsp	sugar	90 mL
½ tsp	ground cinnamon	2 mL
pinch	salt	pinch
2	large eggs	2
1	egg yolk	1
2 cups	2% milk	500 mL
1 tsp	vanilla extract	5 mL

Preheat the oven to 375°F (190°C). Grease six 5 oz (150 mL) baking dishes.

Cut the plums into wedges and arrange them in the baking dishes. In a bowl, combine the flour, sugar, cinnamon, and salt. In a separate bowl, whisk together the eggs, egg yolk, milk, and vanilla. Add the milk mixture to the flour and whisk until combined. Pour this gently over the plums and bake for 25 to 30 minutes, until puffed and golden.

Serve the clafoutis warm or at room temperature with a scoop of ice cream and a drizzle of lavender honey (see left for recipe).

FALL

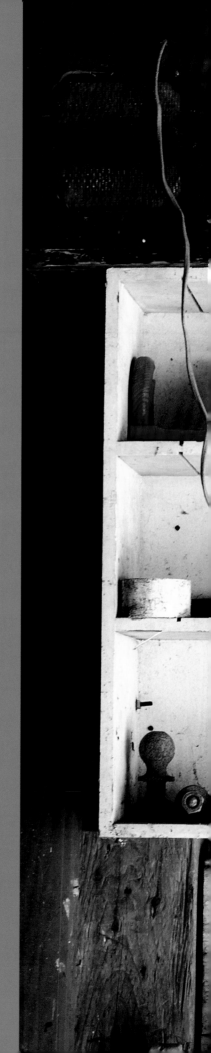

Fall is about the "crackle"—the sound that the leaves make as you kick them while you walk. And maybe, crackle is the sensation of seeing your breath in the air for the first time in months. And crackle is the crisp skin on a roasted chicken, or the crisp skin of a freshly picked apple.

My fashion inclinations and food cravings go hand in hand. I'm just as happy to retire my tank tops and linen pants as I am to retire my need for peaches or blueberries. Out come the sweaters, my old friends, to comfort and warm me while I buy crisp apples and get ready to roast butternut squash.

Every fall I'm amazed by how the foods I'm so tired of by March—onions, apples, potatoes, and broccoli—are suddenly new and exciting again. Who needs strawberries and peaches when I can eat pears and cranberries! Grilling is now the exception and not the rule as I light the pilot in the oven. Fast food is no longer sliced tomatoes and a grilled steak, it's roasted chicken (because all you have to do is pop it in the oven) and apple cranberry crisp.

Bring in the patio furniture, put the fall mums in the garden, and turn on the oven—it's time to make the house smell fabulous!

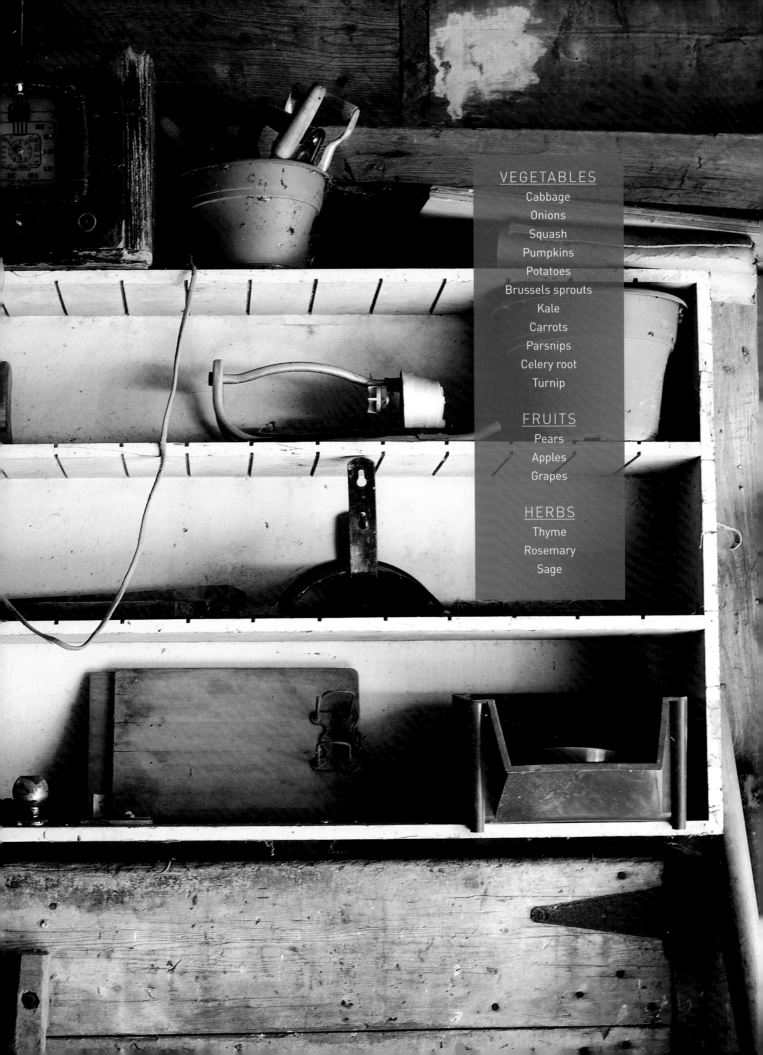

VEGETABLES
Cabbage
Onions
Squash
Pumpkins
Potatoes
Brussels sprouts
Kale
Carrots
Parsnips
Celery root
Turnip

FRUITS
Pears
Apples
Grapes

HERBS
Thyme
Rosemary
Sage

SWEET POTATO SOUP with COCONUT MILK & GINGER *Serves 6*

Silky, sultry, and smooth, this soup plays up the contrast between sweet and heat.

FRESH TAKE

- Figuring out an interesting way to integrate an inherently sweet ingredient into your menu can be challenging. You really need to find a savory application for it. I generally treat sweet potato as I do squash. I sometimes heighten its sweetness with brown sugar or maple syrup when roasting or, in this case, add a touch of hot sauce or chili pepper to build a contrast.

- Like the Spring Pea Soup with Mint (page 5), this soup can be served hot or chilled. It's a refreshing start to a summer supper, but nothing beats it served warm on one of the first brisk days of fall.

- A soup like this is ideal for making ahead and freezing. Nothing of the color, consistency, or taste is the least bit compromised by a month in the freezer.

2 Tbsp	butter	30 mL
1⅓ cups	diced onion	330 mL
6 cups	peeled and diced sweet potato	1.5 L
3–4 cups	chicken stock	750 mL–1 L
1	14 oz (398 mL) can coconut milk	1
2 Tbsp	grated fresh ginger	30 mL
2 Tbsp	fresh lime juice	30 mL
	salt & pepper	
dash	cayenne pepper or hot sauce (optional)	dash
¼ cup	fresh cilantro leaves	60 mL
½ cup	yogurt	125 mL

Melt the butter in a large saucepot over medium heat and cook the onion for 3 to 4 minutes to soften, but not brown. Add the sweet potato, 3 cups (750 mL) of the stock, the coconut milk, and ginger. Simmer for 25 minutes, until the sweet potatoes are tender. Purée the soup with a handheld blender until smooth, adding the remaining stock if too thick, then stir in the lime juice, and strain through a sieve to make it more smooth. Return to the heat and season to taste, including the cayenne or hot sauce, if using.

Ladle the soup into bowls and garnish with cilantro leaves and a swirl of yogurt.

ARUGULA SALAD with
PINEAPPLE, PINE NUTS, & PIAVE *Serves 8*

Color, texture, and taste—three critical elements of a good salad, and they're all in great form here.

FRESH TAKE

• Piave cheese is an Italian pasteurized cow's milk cheese similar to a young Parmesan. It's firm enough to be grated over pasta, or shaved over this salad. I like it here because when you put your nose to the cheese you smell the sweet fragrance of fresh pineapple—seriously!

• I like to serve this salad at the end of a rich fall meal, like a stew or braised dish like Osso Buco (page 110). The subtle bitterness of the greens and the tanginess of the pineapple cleanse the palate, while the buttery pine nuts and Piave cheese combine to mellow everything out.

• To check a pineapple's ripeness, pull at a leaf from the top. If it releases easily, then it's ripe. If you have to tug at it, give the pineapple a day or two on the kitchen counter.

Dressing

3 Tbsp	balsamic vinegar	45 mL
½ tsp	Dijon mustard	2 mL
½ cup	extra virgin olive oil	125 mL
	salt & pepper	

Salad

4 cups	washed arugula	1 L
¼	peeled fresh pineapple	¼
½	red onion	½
⅓ cup	pine nuts, lightly toasted	80 mL
3 oz	Piave cheese (an Italian cheese with the texture of Parmesan, but a lighter, fruity taste)	90 g

For the dressing, whisk the balsamic vinegar with the mustard. Slowly pour in the olive oil while whisking. Season to taste. If the dressing seems thick, whisk in 1 to 2 Tbsp (15 to 30 mL) of water. This will allow the dressing to coat the arugula without weighing it down.

To assemble the salad, arrange the arugula on a serving platter. Remove the core from the pineapple and slice the flesh as thinly as possible (on a mandolin is best). Arrange the pineapple over the arugula. Thinly slice the red onion and arrange it on the salad. Sprinkle the pine nuts overtop. Use a vegetable peeler or cheese knife to peel curls or thin shards of Piave over the salad. Drizzle with the dressing and serve.

MINI SQUASH CHEDDAR SOUFFLÉS with OVEN-ROASTED TOMATOES *Makes 3 dozen mini soufflés*

Hors d'Oeuvre

These soufflés are not the temperature- and time-sensitive beasts that have us cringing at their very mention. Instead, they're light and delicate and impressively easy to make.

FRESH TAKE

- You can skip a step by using 1½ cups (375 mL) of canned pumpkin purée in place of the roasted squash. I recommend this instead of frozen diced butternut squash, which has been blanched and contains too much water to work in this recipe.

- Oven-roasted tomatoes are a contemporary flavor booster. Early fall still boasts beautifully ripe tomatoes, and if you're not the type to home-preserve batches of tomato sauce, roast and then freeze tomatoes in resealable bags—an easy way to later add punch to any pasta sauce. You can also use this roasting technique for Roma tomatoes cut into quarters.

- I first served these at a fundraising event where people "grazed" at each chef's station. I always like to provide a vegetarian option, and I served these alongside the Turkey & Trimmings Pinwheels (page 102). It proved a colorful-looking and tasty table.

1	butternut squash, about ½ lb (250 g)	1
3 Tbsp	unsalted butter	45 mL
3 Tbsp	all-purpose flour	45 mL
1 cup	2% milk	250 mL
1¼ cups	coarsely grated cheddar cheese	310 mL
1 Tbsp	pure maple syrup	15 mL
1 tsp	finely chopped fresh thyme	5 mL
½ tsp	ground nutmeg	2 mL
	salt & pepper	
3	large eggs, separated	3

Preheat the oven to 375°F (190°C). Line a baking tray with parchment paper.

Cut the squash in half lengthwise, scoop out the seeds, and place, flat side down, on the prepared baking tray. Poke holes in the skin of the squash with a fork and bake until tender to the touch, about 35 minutes. Cool, scoop out the squash flesh, and purée until smooth.

Increase the oven temperature to 400°F (200°C). Grease and flour three 12-cup mini muffin tins (36 cups).

Melt the butter in a heavy-bottomed saucepot over medium heat, then add the flour and cook, stirring with a wooden spoon, for 2 minutes. Whisk in the milk in a slow stream, bring to a full simmer whisking constantly, and cook until thickened, about 4 minutes. Reduce the heat to low then stir in the cheese until it melts. Remove the pot from the heat and stir in the puréed squash, maple syrup, thyme, and nutmeg and season to taste. Stir in the egg yolks.

Whip the egg whites until they hold a medium peak when the beaters are lifted. Fold half the whites into the squash mixture until just incorporated, then fold in the remaining half. Spoon or pipe the mixture into the prepared mini muffin cups to three-quarters full. Bake for 15 to 18 minutes, until soufflés have puffed up and are golden on top. They will fall about a minute after they come out of the oven.

Serve the soufflés warm or at room temperature, with an oven-roasted grape tomato on top. If preparing ahead of time, store soufflés refrigerated for up to 2 days, and re-warm on a baking tray in a 300°F (150°C) oven.

OVEN-ROASTED TOMATOES

Makes about 1 cup (250 ml)

1 pint / 2 cups	ripe grape tomatoes	500 mL
2 Tbsp	olive oil	30 mL
2 tsp	sugar	10 mL
½ tsp	coarse salt	2 mL
¼ tsp	ground black pepper	1 mL

Preheat the oven to 225°F (105°C). Line a baking tray with parchment paper.

Cut the tomatoes in half and place them, cut side up, on the prepared baking tray (close together is just fine). Drizzle them with the olive oil, sprinkle them with the sugar, salt, and pepper and roast them until they're no longer juicy but not browned, about 75 minutes. Cool and store refrigerated until ready to use.

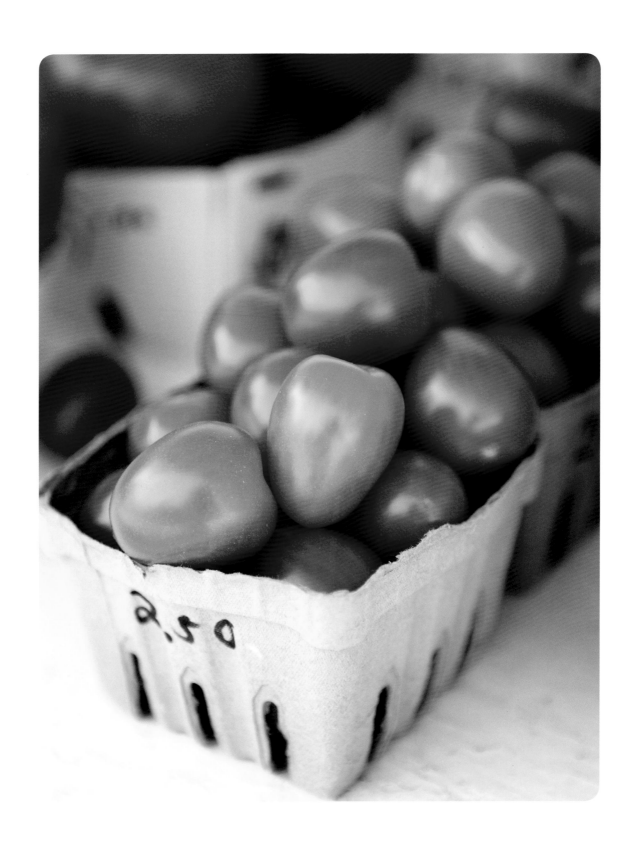

SPELT CRUST PIZZA with ARTICHOKES & MUSHROOMS *Makes two 9-inch (23 cm) pizzas*

This "white pizza," with its thin crust and lively toppings, is one of my personal favorites.

FRESH TAKE

- Spelt flour is lower in gluten than wheat flour, but it's not gluten free. It's a good choice for a thin-crust pizza because the lower gluten makes for more of a crispy, crackerlike crust that's easy to roll out.

- My little trick is to stir some sour cream into the pesto for the pizza sauce. I find that sometimes pesto on its own is either too dry or too oily. The sour cream holds the pesto in place and adds a nice bit of moisture.

- A hot oven is crucial to a properly cooked pizza. A pizza stone is a good investment if you like making pizza at home. Placing the pizza on a preheated stone instantly brings the yeast in the crust to life. The yeast forms tiny bubbles that toast up and give the pizza the perfect crackle, and enough structure to hold up under the toppings.

Spelt Pizza Dough

¾ cup	tepid water (105°F/41°C)	185 mL
2¼ tsp	(1 pkg) instant dry yeast	11 mL
1 cup	all-purpose flour	250 mL
1 cup	spelt flour	250 mL
3 Tbsp	olive oil	45 mL
1 tsp	salt	5 mL

Toppings

2 Tbsp	olive oil	30 mL
½ lb	cremini mushrooms, sliced	250 g
2 cloves	garlic, minced	2 cloves
1	14 oz (398 mL) jar marinated artichokes	1
1 tsp	lemon zest	5 mL
	salt & pepper	
¼ cup	basil pesto	60 mL
3 Tbsp	sour cream (not low-fat)	45 mL
	cornmeal, for sprinkling	
8–12 slices	prosciutto ham	8–12 slices
2 oz	Parmesan	60 g
⅓ cup	loosely packed fresh basil leaves	80 mL
2 cups	loosely packed baby arugula leaves	500 mL

For the dough, stir together the water and yeast, then stir in the flours, olive oil, and salt until the dough becomes difficult to work with a wooden spoon. Turn it out onto a lightly floured surface and knead for just 1 minute, until it feels elastic. Place the dough in a lightly oiled bowl, cover with plastic wrap, and let it rest at room temperature for 30 minutes.

Meanwhile, prepare the toppings. In a large sauté pan over medium heat add the olive oil. Add the mushrooms and sauté them until tender, about 5 minutes. Add the garlic and stir. Add the artichokes and lemon zest, warm through, and season to taste. In a small bowl, stir together the pesto and sour cream.

Preheat the oven to 500°F (260°C). Place a baking tray or pizza stone in the oven.

Continued . . .

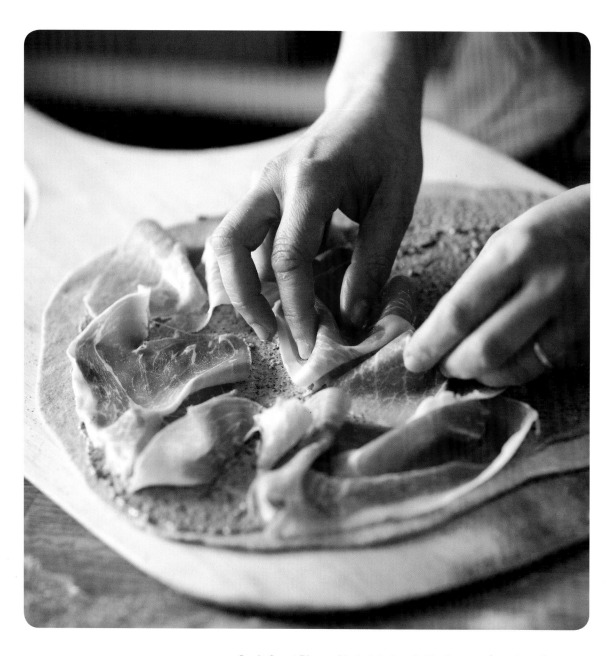

Spelt Crust Pizza with Artichokes & Mushrooms (continued)

Divide the dough into 2 pieces and, on a lightly floured surface, roll out each piece as thinly as possible to about 9 inches (23 cm) across. Remove the hot pan from the oven and sprinkle it lightly with cornmeal. Place the first rolled crust on the pan and spread it all over with a thin layer of the pesto mixture. Arrange half the prosciutto on top, spoon over half the mushroom-artichoke filling, and bake for 10 to 15 minutes, until the pizza is golden at the edges. Slide the pizza off the pan and repeat with the second crust.

Grate Parmesan over the cooked pizzas with a vegetable peeler, and top with basil leaves and arugula immediately before serving.

MISO GRILLED EGGPLANT & SCALLOPS

Serves 6 as an appetizer, 4 as an entrée

This dish suits fall because of the earthy richness that the miso glaze provides. This can be served as an entrée or a starter course.

½ cup	light miso paste (found at Asian food stores or health food stores)	125 mL
2 Tbsp	honey	30 mL
2 Tbsp	mirin or sake	30 mL
2	Japanese eggplants	2
1 lb	large sea scallops (dry-pack frozen)	500 g
1 Tbsp	lightly toasted sesame seeds	15 mL

For the glaze, stir together the first three ingredients and chill until ready to use.

Preheat the grill to high heat.

Slice the eggplant on the bias into ½-inch-thick (1 cm) pieces. Grill them until they're soft and showing grill marks, about 3 minutes, then turn them over. Brush the glaze on the cooked side of the eggplants, then turn over again to cook for 1 minute more on the first side while glazing the second side. Turn over to cook the glaze on the second side. Remove the eggplant from the grill and set it aside on a platter. Use this same method with the scallops, cooking for about 6 minutes in total.

Serve the eggplant and scallops warm and garnished with sesame seeds.

TURKEY ESCALOPE *Serves 4*

This French version of schnitzel offers an unconventional means to serve turkey.

FRESH TAKE

· Escalopes, or thin slices, of turkey are easy to do because of the larger size of the turkey breast. You can also purchase the escalope already done for you, typically sold in groceries as *scaloppine*.

· Because of its simplicity, I like to serve turkey escalope with more interesting sides, such as the Swiss chard dish on page 115 and the roasted root vegetables on page 118.

· Safe food handling is always important, but it's particularly worth mentioning here as turkey is a bacterial culprit. prit. Be sure to use a clean set of tongs to remove the cooked turkey from the pan, and, of course, sanitize any tools or surfaces that may have come in contact with the turkey before it was cooked.

1	2 lb (1 kg) turkey breast, on the bone	1
	salt & pepper	
¾ cup	all-purpose flour	185 mL
2	eggs	2
¼ cup	cold 2% milk	60 mL
1 cup	dry breadcrumbs	250 mL
1 tsp	finely chopped fresh thyme	5 mL
2 Tbsp	butter	30 mL
2 Tbsp	olive oil	30 mL
	juice of 1 lemon	

Use a sharp knife to take the turkey breast off the bone. Slice the turkey in half against the grain, then slice each half into 2 thin slices. Place 1 slice inside a resealable bag, and pound with a meat tenderizer until thin but without tearing the meat (or the bag). Repeat with the 3 remaining slices.

To prepare the turkey for breading, stir a little salt and pepper into the flour in a shallow bowl. Whisk the eggs with the milk in another shallow bowl and season lightly. Season the breadcrumbs lightly and mix them with the thyme in a third flat bowl.

Preheat a large sauté pan over medium-high heat and melt 1 Tbsp (15 mL) of the butter and 1 Tbsp (15 mL) of the oil. Dip a turkey escalope in the flour, coating both sides. Shake off any excess flour then dip the escalope into the egg mixture, coating well again. Shake off any excess then coat it completely in breadcrumbs. Add the escalope to the skillet and repeat with the other escalopes. You can fill the pan but don't crowd it. Cook the escalopes for about 4 minutes on each side, until cooked through. Place the cooked cutlets on a platter or baking tray and keep them warm in a 325°F (160°C) oven. Add the remaining butter and oil to the skillet and cook remaining escalopes.

Squeeze over lemon juice immediately before serving.

The turkey escalopes can be breaded and refrigerated for up to 2 hours before cooking.

Poultry

WHOLE ROASTED PORK LOIN with ONIONS, PEARS, & ORANGE *Serves 6 to 8*

I love a good roast in the fall. Fall is the beginning of comfort food season, and filling the house with the fragrances of home-cooking is incredibly soothing.

FRESH TAKE

- Move over grilling season and barbecue sauce—it's time for oven roasting and basting glazes. Because the marmalade in the glaze is somewhat diluted by the other ingredients, the glaze can be applied before the pork goes in the oven. It won't scorch, just caramelize slightly.

- The sauce for this pork roast is simpler to make than a gravy. The glaze that drips off the roast as it cooks serves to thicken the sauce, so there's no need for flour or cornstarch to achieve a proper sauce consistency.

- I'm a big fan of the orange and pear combination, but you could easily use apples and lemons, or dried apricots and limes.

Pork

2	medium onions, peeled and sliced	2
½ cup	grainy mustard	125 mL
3 Tbsp	orange marmalade	45 mL
2 Tbsp	unsalted butter, at room temperature	30 mL
1 Tbsp	salt	15 mL
1 tsp	ground black pepper	5 mL
3 lb	boneless pork loin roast	1.5 kg
2	Bartlett pears, cored and sliced	2
1	orange, unpeeled and quartered	1
3 sprigs	fresh thyme	3 sprigs
1 sprig	fresh sage	1 sprig

Pan Sauce

½ cup	dry white wine	125 mL
1 cup	chicken stock	250 mL
1 tsp	finely chopped fresh sage	5 mL
3 Tbsp	cold unsalted butter	45 mL
	salt & pepper	

Preheat the oven to 375°F (190°C).

In a food processor, purée half the onion slices, and the grainy mustard, marmalade, butter, salt, and pepper. Place the pork roast (it can be tied or untied) in a roasting pan and slather it with the mustard glaze. Arrange the remaining onion slices, pears, orange, and fresh herbs around the pork loin. Roast the pork, uncovered, for 15 minutes, then reduce the oven temperature to 350°F (180°C), roasting for about 75 minutes, until an internal temperature of 175°F (80°C) is reached. Remove the roast from the pan and let it rest on a cutting board or platter for 15 minutes before slicing.

For the pan sauce, remove the orange segments and thyme and sage sprigs from the pan and discard them. Place the pan over medium heat and add the white wine, stirring to pull up any caramelized bits from the bottom of the pan. Add the chicken stock and fresh sage and simmer until reduced by half. Reduce the heat to low and stir in the cold butter just until melted. Season to taste and serve alongside slices of roast pork.

Meat

OSSO BUCO *Serves 8*

Luscious and rich, this Italian classic is a personal favorite, especially when I'm entertaining. Serve it with the gremolata and saffron acini di pepe (page 113) for the perfect Italian meal.

FRESH TAKE

· A braised dish is ideal for entertaining as the work is all done in advance. And if your guests are running late, or you're enjoying chatting and nibbling on hors d'oeuvres and don't want to rush the pace, a braised dish will happily sit and wait for you, uncompromised.

· Gremolata (see page 112) is a piquant accompaniment for osso buco that cuts its richness. Serve just a small spoonful on top of the osso buco, and stir it in a little as you take a bite.

· The olives are best stirred in at the very end of cooking. If you add them near the beginning of the long braising process they could add some bitterness to the sauce.

4 Tbsp	olive oil, divided	60 mL
6 lb	veal shank pieces (about 1 large or 2 small per person)	2.7 kg
4 cups	diced onion	1 L
2 cups	diced celery	500 mL
2 cups	peeled and diced carrot	500 mL
3 cloves	garlic, crushed	3 cloves
1½ cups	dry white wine	375 mL
2	28 oz (796 mL) cans diced tomato	2
4 sprigs	fresh thyme	4 sprigs
4 sprigs	fresh oregano	4 sprigs
2	bay leaves	2
1 cup	kalamata olives	250 mL
	salt & pepper	

Preheat the oven to 325°F (160°C).

Heat a large ovenproof pot over medium-high heat and add 1 Tbsp (15 mL) of the oil. Sear the veal shanks on each side until browned. Remove them from the pan and set aside. You may have to do this in batches, adding more oil after each batch.

Reduce the heat to medium and add the onion, celery, and carrot, sautéing until the onion is translucent, about 5 minutes. Add the garlic and cook for 1 minute more. Stir in the white wine, bring it to a simmer, then add the tomatoes. Stir in the thyme, oregano, and bay leaves. Return the veal shanks to the pot, ensuring they're covered with liquid (add water if necessary). Bring the liquid to a simmer, cover the pot, then transfer it to the oven. Cook for 2 to 2½ hours, until the veal pulls away from the bone easily.

You may keep it warm in a 275°F (140°C) oven until you are ready to serve, or if prepared beforehand, reheat it in a 325°F (160°C) oven. To serve, place the veal on a serving plate. Remove the herbs from the pot and return the sauce to a simmer. Stir in the olives and adjust the seasoning. Spoon sauce over the veal and serve with a spoonful of gremolata.

Continued . . .

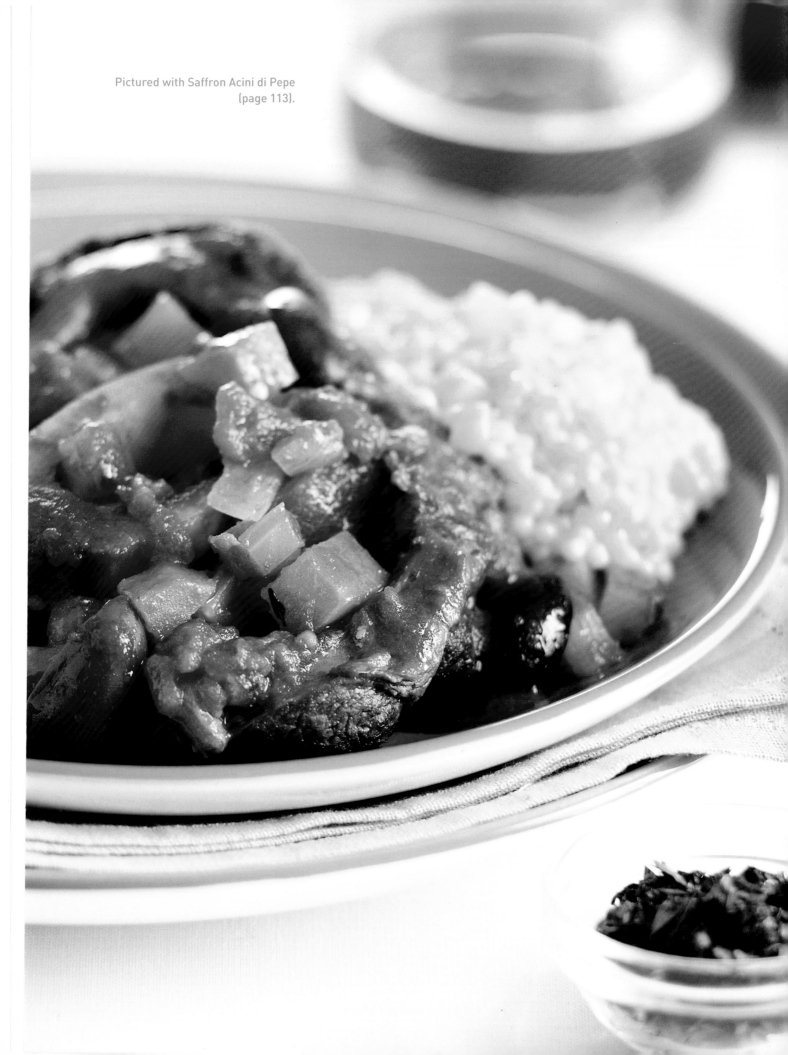

Pictured with Saffron Acini di Pepe
(page 113).

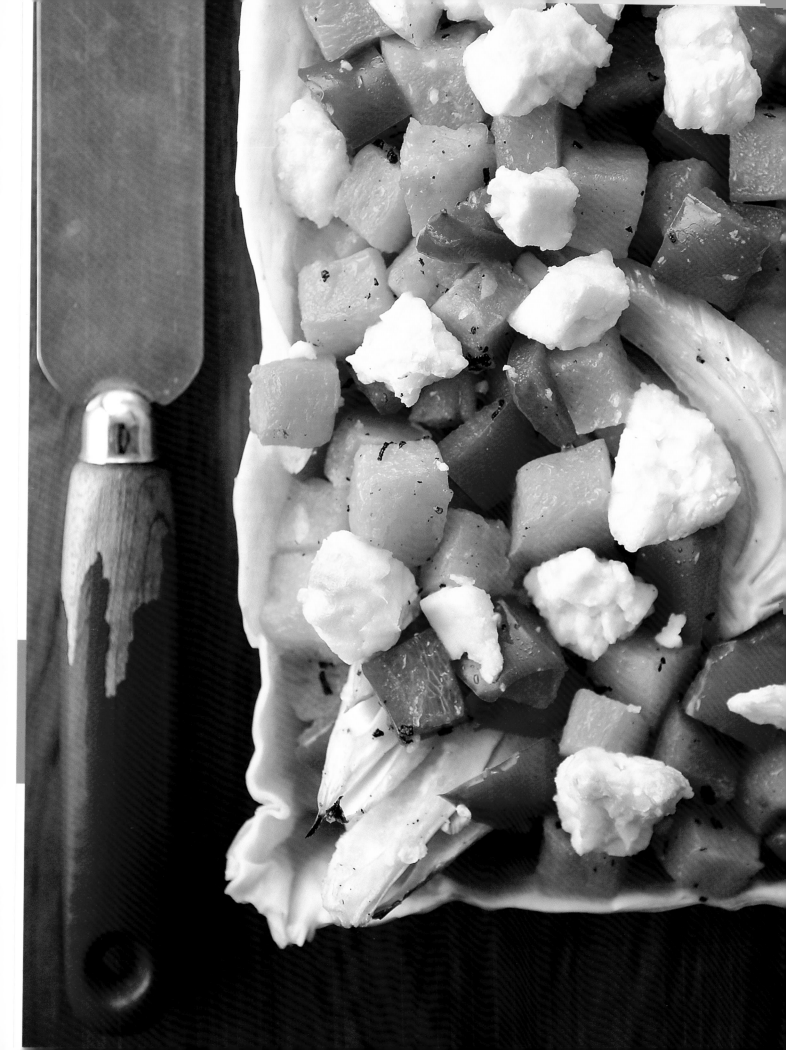

ROASTED VEGETABLE TART *Serves 6*

A creative way to serve your veggies! I like to offer this alongside roasted chicken or pork, or even as a nice appetizer course.

FRESH TAKE

- Peeling the garlic and poaching it in oil is a real chef's trick for roasting garlic. This way the garlic cloves are evenly roasted (and can be puréed and frozen), the oil becomes garlic infused, and you don't have the mess of squishing out garlic from the head.

- Use any leftover garlic oil to baste a chicken or pork roast, toss with potatoes for roasting, or make a roasted garlic vinaigrette.

- Make sure your oven is preheated to 375°F (190°C) before you put in the tart so that the phyllo crusts up and browns on the bottom.

Roasted Garlic Oil

1 head	garlic	1 head
1 cup	canola oil	250 mL

Vegetable Tart

6 cups	peeled and diced butternut squash	1.5 L
	salt & pepper	
1	red bell pepper, diced	1
½ head	sliced fennel	½ head
1 Tbsp	finely chopped fresh sage	15 mL
1 tsp	finely grated lemon zest	5 mL
3 sheets	phyllo pastry	3 sheets
4 oz	feta cheese	125 g

Preheat the oven to 375°F (190°C).

For the roasted garlic and oil, peel the garlic cloves and place them in a baking dish. Cover with oil, stir to coat, and cover the dish. Bake until the garlic cloves are golden, about 40 minutes. Let cool and spoon out garlic for later use. (Only the oil will be used for this recipe.)

Toss the squash with 3 Tbsp (45 mL) of the garlic oil and season it lightly. Bake the squash, covered, for 15 minutes at 375°F (190°C). Reduce the oven temperature to 350°F (180°C), and bake, uncovered, until the squash is tender, about 20 more minutes.

Toss the cooled squash with the diced bell pepper, sliced fennel, sage, and lemon zest. Season to taste.

To assemble the tart, increase the oven temperature to 375°F (190°C) again. Spread out 1 sheet of phyllo (keeping the other sheets covered). Brush it lightly with garlic oil, lay the second sheet on top, and brush the second sheet with garlic oil. Repeat with the third sheet. Fold the phyllo in half lengthwise then gently transfer it to an ungreased 4- × 10-inch (10 × 25 cm) tart pan with a removable bottom. Spoon vegetable filling into the tart shell and crumble the feta overtop. Bake for 20 to 25 minutes, until the phyllo is a rich brown.

Serve the tart warm or at room temperature.

Vegetables

ROASTED ROOT VEGETABLES with WARM VINAIGRETTE *Serves 6*

A warm vinaigrette adds sparkle to a dish expected to be served as part of a fall supper. There's no better combination than carrots, parsnips, celery root, and squash for dinner after a day of raking leaves or carving pumpkins.

FRESH TAKE

- While some of these root vegetables take longer to cook than others (celery root takes the least time and carrot the most), none of them are compromised by being cooked for longer. Use the carrot as the measure for doneness.

- Delicata squash looks like a zucchini with green and yellow zebra stripes, and like a zucchini, its skin is edible, although the seeds are more like a butternut's and need to be scooped out. If you can't get your hands on Delicata, peeled and diced butternut or Hubbard squash would work just fine.

- The warm vinaigrette can also be used as a sauce for roasted chicken in lieu of gravy, or spooned over a spinach salad with apple slices and onion.

Roasted Root Vegetables

1 cup	peeled and diced carrot	250 mL
1 cup	peeled and diced parsnip	250 mL
1 cup	diced celery root	250 mL
1	Delicata squash, cut in half lengthwise, seeded, and diced	1
2	shallots, sliced	2
3 Tbsp	olive oil	45 mL
2 sprigs	fresh thyme	2 sprigs
	salt & pepper	

Warm Vinaigrette

1 + 6 Tbsp	olive oil	15 + 90 mL
1	shallot, minced	1
2 Tbsp	apple cider vinegar	30 mL
1 tsp	Dijon mustard	5 mL
1 tsp	finely chopped fresh rosemary	5 mL
	salt & pepper	
2 Tbsp	roasted pumpkin seeds	30 mL

Preheat the oven to 350°F (180°C).

Toss the carrot, parsnip, celery root, and squash with the shallots, olive oil, and thyme and season lightly. Place the vegetables in an 8-cup (2 L) baking dish and roast for 30 to 40 minutes, until they're equally tender. Remove the thyme.

For the vinaigrette, heat 1 Tbsp (15 mL) of the oil and sauté the shallot for 1 minute over medium heat. Whisk in the vinegar, mustard, and rosemary and reduce the heat to low. Whisk in the remaining oil in a slow drizzle and season to taste.

Toss the warm roasted vegetables with the warm vinaigrette, garnish with the pumpkin seeds, and serve immediately.

Vegetables

FRUIT & NUT MUESLI *Serves 4*

Unlike cereal that gets mushy and icky if it sits in milk, muesli, soaked in yogurt and fruit, improves as it sits in the fridge.

FRESH TAKE

· It's important to use regular rolled oats and not instant here. The nut and grain mixture softens up as it sits in the fruit and yogurt mixture, and instant oats would absorb the liquid too quickly, making the muesli stodgy instead of just soft.

· This is one of those "tailor your own" recipes—add all berries if you wish, or use sliced peaches or pineapple . . . it's up to you. The combo here is simply my preference.

· Every year Michael and I travel to a fabulous lodge in the Rockies in November for a food and wine event. Outside of the obvious pleasures like the scenic vistas and large blazing fireplaces, I look forward to their remarkable breakfast buffet. It is their muesli that has inspired me to create this concoction.

1 cup	rolled oats (not instant)	250 mL
⅓ cup	sliced almonds	80 mL
¼ cup	untoasted wheat germ	60 mL
¼ cup	spelt or barley flakes (found at health or bulk food stores)	60 mL
2 Tbsp	unsalted roasted pumpkin seeds	30 mL
1 Tbsp	sesame seeds	15 mL
⅓ cup	raisins	80 mL
2 cups	yogurt	500 mL
2 Tbsp	honey or maple syrup	30 mL
1	small apple, peeled and coarsely grated	1
1	small banana, diced (frozen is fine)	1
1 cup	diced strawberries	250 mL

Preheat the oven to 350°F (180°C). Line a baking tray with parchment paper.

Measure the oats, almonds, wheat germ, and spelt or barley onto the prepared tray and stir to mix. Toast for 12 minutes, stirring once, and cool.

Pour the cooled mixture into a medium bowl and stir in the remaining ingredients. Cover and chill for at least 4 hours or overnight.

HONEY OAT ROASTED PEARS *Serves 6*

Love baked apples? These pears are an elegant variation that I like to serve warm in the morning in place of oatmeal (though I do love my oatmeal!).

FRESH TAKE

· If after cutting the pears in half and coring them they don't sit flat in the baking dish, slice a flat spot on the underside of the pear.

· I find pears of medium ripeness work best for oven roasting. Too firm and they won't soften up, too ripe and they just turn squishy. The pear should just give a little when pressed gently.

· Okay, I'll let you get away with this as dessert too. I've done it before and served the pears warm with a scoop of vanilla ice cream, drizzling the honey over the ice cream too.

1 cup	rolled oats	250 mL
⅓ cup	packed light brown sugar	80 mL
¼ cup	sliced almonds	60 mL
½ tsp	ground cinnamon	2 mL
¼ cup	unsalted butter, melted, plus extra for brushing	60 mL
3 Tbsp	raisins	45 mL
4	Bartlett or Bosc Pears	4
	honey, for drizzling	

Preheat the oven to 375°F (190°C).

Toss the oats, brown sugar, almonds, and cinnamon to combine. Stir in the melted butter until everything is roughly combined. Stir in the raisins. Cut the pears in half (don't peel them) and scoop out their cores. Lay the pear halves in a baking dish and brush their tops with more melted butter. Press some oat filling into the center of each pear. Bake, uncovered, for 25 minutes, until the pears are tender and the oat filling is lightly browned.

Serve warm, drizzled with honey, and with yogurt on the side if desired.

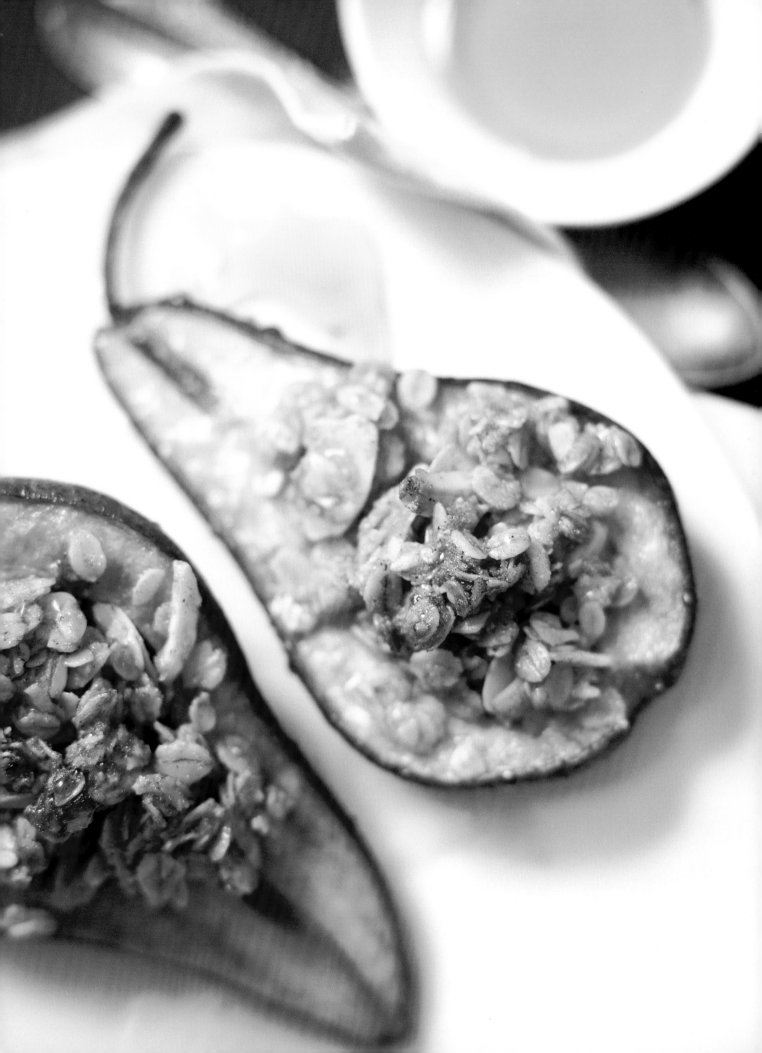

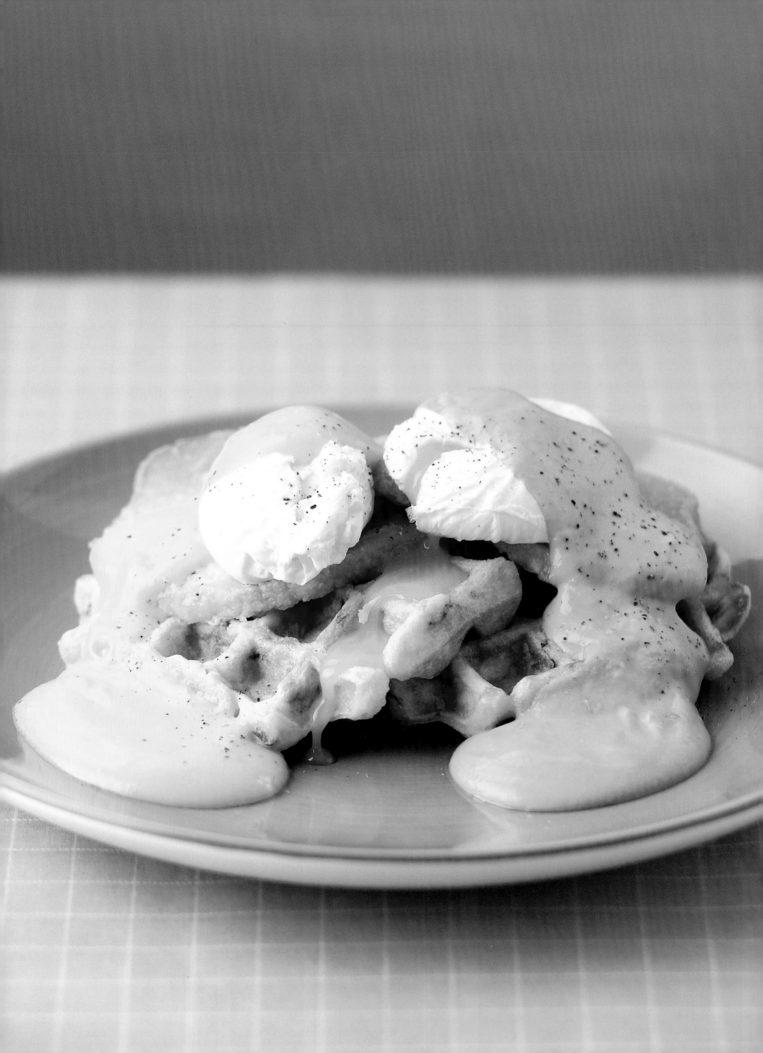

EGGS BENEDICT with PEAMEAL & TOMATO "CREAM" on SCALLION WAFFLES

Makes 8 to 10 waffles • Serves 4

This is a special recipe for a special occasion. In place of a traditional hollandaise, I make a fresh, creamy tomato sauce, and in place of English muffins, savory waffles whose crevices embrace every bit of tasty goodness.

FRESH TAKE

- The tomato "cream" is a trick I picked up from Michael. The acidity of the tomatoes emulsifies, or binds, with the oil, creating a sauce with the consistency of a thin mayonnaise and a full fresh tomato taste. I find cherry or grape tomatoes work much better than regular tomatoes. Try this on your next BLT in place of mayo!

- Waffles are no more difficult to make than pancakes, so if you have a waffle iron, pull it out of the cupboard and put it to use!

- Poaching eggs, on the other hand, is a real art. Twirling the water to create a whirlpool and adding vinegar both help to keep the egg white from going all over the place. This creates the oval shape that, once cooked, is easy to lift out of the water with a slotted spoon.

SCALLION WAFFLES

2 cups	all-purpose flour	500 mL
2 Tbsp	cornmeal	30 mL
2 tsp	baking powder	10 mL
1 tsp	salt	5 mL
½ tsp	baking soda	2 mL
2	eggs	2
2 cups	buttermilk	500 mL
½ cup	unsalted butter, melted	125 mL
1 cup	finely chopped scallions (green onions)	250 mL
	oil, for greasing waffle iron	

Stir the flour, cornmeal, baking powder, salt, and baking soda to combine. In a separate bowl, whisk together the eggs, buttermilk, and melted butter. Add this buttermilk mixture to the flour mixture and stir just until blended. Stir in the scallions.

Preheat a waffle iron and lightly grease it. Make the waffles according to the manufacturer's instructions (about ⅓ cup (80 mL) batter for a standard waffle) and keep warm in a 250°F (120°C) oven until ready to serve.

Continued . . .

TOMATO "CREAM"

Makes 2 cups (500 ml)

1 pint / 2 cups	ripe cherry or grape tomatoes	500 mL
½ cup	canola or grapeseed oil	125 mL
	salt & pepper	

Wash the tomatoes then place them in a jar and purée finely with an immersion blender. While blending, gradually pour in the oil. The mixture will emulsify and look like a tomato mayonnaise. Strain the sauce through a sieve, season to taste, and chill until ready to serve.

For a twist, this recipe can be made using red, orange, *and* yellow tomatoes. Blend each tomato color separately with oil, then strain through a sieve.

POACHED EGGS WITH PEAMEAL

8 slices	peameal bacon, cooked	8 slices
1 Tbsp	white vinegar	15 mL
8	large eggs	8

Keep the peameal warm while you prepare the eggs.

Fill a pot with 16 cups (4 L) water, add the vinegar, and bring to just below a simmer. Break an egg into a cup. Stir the water to create a "whirlpool" in its center. Drop the egg just to the side of the center (the water should still be moving) and cook it until set on the outside but the yolk is still visibly soft (for "easy"), about 4 minutes. You can cook the eggs 2 or 3 at a time. Remove them from the water with a slotted spoon.

To assemble this dish, place 2 waffles on a plate and arrange a slice of peameal bacon on each. Top with poached eggs and spoon tomato cream over. Serve immediately.

COUNTRY APPLE PIE *Makes one 9-inch (23 cm) pie*

I make this at home at least once a year just because it's the perfect way to celebrate fall.

FRESH TAKE

- This crust is my staple pie pastry recipe. I've also featured it in the baby cherry pies recipe on page 86. The balance of butter and shortening creates a crust that is tender, tasty, and flaky without getting soggy (the shortening at work), and melts in your mouth (the butter factor).

- Too often we're warned not to add too much water to a pie dough. We become afraid and don't add enough. When you start rolling the dough, if the crust immediately begins to crack, it means it needs water. Simply dip your fingers in cold water and sprinkle it over the half-rolled dough. Gather the dough, kneading it for just a moment to work in the water, and chill for 1 hour before rolling again . . . perfect!

- Ah, the choice of apples. This topic is often debated here in my part of the country, which grows over a dozen types of apples. What seems to come up the most in discussions is that a combination of apples is the winning factor. And I should know winning pies. I had to judge an apple pie contest a year back and there were 60 entrants! If I recall correctly, the top three pies all contained a blend of apple varieties.

Pastry

2½ cups	all-purpose flour	625 mL
½ tsp	fine sea salt	2 mL
½ cup	cold unsalted butter, cut into pieces	125 mL
½ cup	cold vegetable shortening, cut into pieces	125 mL
2 Tbsp	lemon juice	30 mL
4–8 Tbsp	cold water	60–125 mL

Filling

8 cups	peeled, cored, and sliced tart apples, such as Northern Spy or Spartan or a mix	2 L
¾ cup	sugar	185 mL
½ cup	packed light brown sugar	125 mL
2 Tbsp	all-purpose flour	30 mL
1 tsp	finely grated lemon zest	5 mL
1 Tbsp	lemon juice	15 mL
1 tsp	ground cinnamon	5 mL
¼ tsp	ground nutmeg	1 mL
2 Tbsp	unsalted butter	30 mL
1	egg whisked with 2 Tbsp (30 mL) cold water, for brushing	1
	sugar, for sprinkling	

For the pastry, combine the flour with the salt. Cut in the butter and shortening until the mixture has a roughly even crumbly texture. Add the lemon juice and cold water—begin with 4 Tbsp (60 mL) water and add more if necessary, 1 Tbsp (15 mL) at a time—and blend just until the dough comes together. Shape into a disk, then wrap it and chill for 30 minutes.

For the filling, toss together the apples, both sugars, flour, lemon zest and juice, cinnamon, and nutmeg and set aside.

Preheat the oven to 400°F (200°C). On a lightly floured surface, roll out half the dough to just under ¼ inch (6 mm) thick. Lightly dust the bottom of a 9-inch (23 cm) pie pan with flour and line the pan with the dough. Fill the pastry with the apples and dot the top with the butter. Roll out the remaining dough and place over the apples. Trim and cinch the edges of the pie and cut holes in the top to let steam escape. Brush with egg wash and sprinkle lightly with sugar. Bake for 10 minutes, then reduce the heat to 375°F (190°C) and bake for about another 40 minutes, until the filling is bubbling. Let the pie cool for at least 1 hour before slicing.

SPICED CHOCOLATE PEAR TART

Makes one 9-inch (23 cm) tart

Pears and chocolate are a divine combination. Think Belle Hélène, a classic French dessert of a poached pear filled with chocolate ganache and served with a custard sauce.

FRESH TAKE

- It's important to place a piece of parchment paper on the surface of the poaching liquid while the pears cook. Part of the pears float above the poaching liquid, and the liquid gently hits the parchment and flows over the pears so that they cook evenly. Without the paper, you'd have a firm spot on every pear.

- Making this tart crust is just like making cookie dough. It's easy to handle, but it does need some chilling time so the butter sets enough to roll easily.

- The pastry and filling is a twist on the French *tarte au chocolat*. The addition of cinnamon, cardamom, and black pepper gives it a nice lick, keeping it from tasting too sweet.

Pears

3	Anjou or Bartlett pears, peeled, halved, and cored	3
2 cups	sugar	500 mL
1 Tbsp	lemon juice	15 mL
2 Tbsp	brandy	30 mL

Crust

½ cup	unsalted butter, at room temperature	125 mL
3 Tbsp	sugar	45 mL
2	large egg yolks	2
¾ cup	all-purpose flour	185 mL
¼ cup	cocoa powder	60 mL
½ tsp	fine sea salt	2 mL

Filling

6 oz	bittersweet or semisweet chocolate, chopped	175 g
¾ cup	whipping cream	185 mL
1 tsp	ground cinnamon	5 mL
½ tsp	ground cardamom	2 mL
¼ tsp	ground black pepper	1 mL
1 tsp	vanilla extract	5 mL
1	large egg	1

Bring the pears, sugar, 2 cups (500 mL) water, and lemon juice up to a simmer. Place a piece of parchment (or a plate) directly on the surface of the liquid to keep the pears from floating. Cook the pears at just below a simmer until just tender, about 10 minutes. Remove from the heat. After the pears have cooled completely, remove them from the poaching liquid, sprinkle with the brandy, toss, and chill until ready to serve. Discard the poaching liquid.

For the crust, cream together the butter and sugar. Add the egg yolks one at a time, stirring after each addition. Sift together the flour, cocoa, and salt and add this to the butter mixture. Mix until the dough just comes together. Shape it into a disk and chill until you're ready to roll. If preparing ahead of time, pull the dough from the fridge an hour before rolling.

On a lightly floured surface, roll out the dough to just over ¼ inch (6 mm) thick. Line a 9-inch (23 cm) tart pan with a removable bottom with the dough, trim the edges, and chill for 20 minutes.

Preheat the oven to 350°F (180°C).

Dock the pastry with a fork and bake for 18 to 20 minutes. Allow to cool.

Reduce the oven temperature to 325°F (160°C).

Place the chopped chocolate in a large bowl. In a pot, heat the cream with the dry spices to just below a simmer and then pour over the chocolate. Let this sit for a minute then stir slowly until smooth. Stir in the vanilla. Whisk the egg in a small cup then stir it into the chocolate. Pour this into the chocolate shell and bake for 12 minutes. Let cool for 15 minutes then chill for at least 2 hours before serving.

To serve, slice the pears thinly and arrange over the tart.

PUMPKIN CRÈME BRÛLÉE *Serves 8*

Pumpkin pie without the fuss of making a crust!

FRESH TAKE

- It's important to use pie pumpkins for roasting and not the décor pumpkins you carve out for Halloween—they're too stringy and watery. Pie pumpkins are smaller and rounder and have darker skin to them, and their flesh is creamy and smooth once cooked and puréed. If you're pressed for time, you can also use 2 cups (500 mL) of canned pumpkin purée.

- The key difference between this recipe and a pumpkin pie filling is the use of more egg yolks and cream here. A crème brûlée needs to have that custard character to it.

- I like to brûlée my custards with turbinado sugar, a dry, coarse style of brown sugar. It has a caramel taste and melts into a nice thick layer on top. It's not the end of the world if you have only regular granulated sugar, though. Just sprinkle and (carefully) torch the sugar repeating a few times to build thin layers, which will eventually become a nice thick caramel crust, worthy of a good smack with the back of a spoon.

1–2	small pie pumpkins	1–2
2½ cups	whipping cream	625 mL
1	vanilla bean	1
½ cup	packed light brown sugar	125 mL
10	large egg yolks	10
2 Tbsp	granulated sugar	30 mL
½ tsp + ¼ tsp	ground cinnamon	2 mL + 1 mL
½ tsp	ground ginger	2 mL
¼ tsp	ground allspice	1 mL
1 Tbsp	brandy	15 mL
½ cup	turbinado sugar, for brûlée	125 mL

Preheat the oven to 350°F (180°C). Line a baking tray with parchment paper.

Cut the pumpkins in half, scoop out and discard the seeds, and place the pumpkins cut side down on the prepared baking tray. Dock the pumpkin surfaces with a fork and bake for 30 to 40 minutes, until tender. Cool then scoop out the pumpkin flesh and purée until smooth. Measure out 2 cups (500 mL) for the crème brûlée and refrigerate or freeze the remainder for use in soup or pumpkin pie.

Reduce the oven temperature to 325°F (160°C). Place eight 5 oz (150 mL) ramekins in a baking dish with a 2-inch (5 cm) lip.

Heat the whipping cream with seeds scraped out of the vanilla bean until just below a simmer. In a food processor, combine the egg yolks, granulated sugar, ½ tsp (2 mL) of the cinnamon, and the ginger, allspice, and brandy with the reserved 2 cups (500 mL) of pumpkin. Pour the hot cream into the pumpkin mixture and combine. Pour this custard into the ramekins and fill the baking pan with hot tap water (rest the pan on the oven door to make it easier). Bake for 30 to 35 minutes, until the custards are set but jiggle just slightly in the center. Remove the custards from the pan, cool for 20 minutes, then chill for at least 4 hours.

To brûlée the custards, toss the remaining ¼ tsp (1 mL) cinnamon with the turbinado sugar. Sprinkle it onto the custards, and caramelize them with a butane torch (available at kitchen supply stores). Chill the brûlées for up to 2 hours or serve immediately.

Sweets

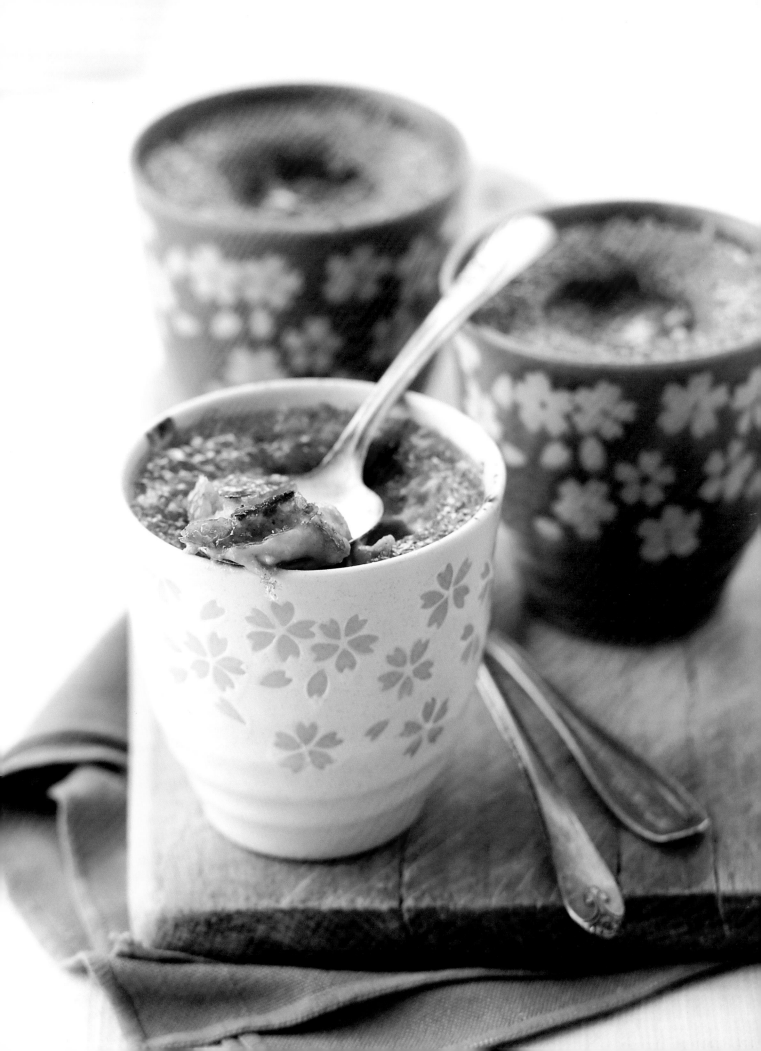

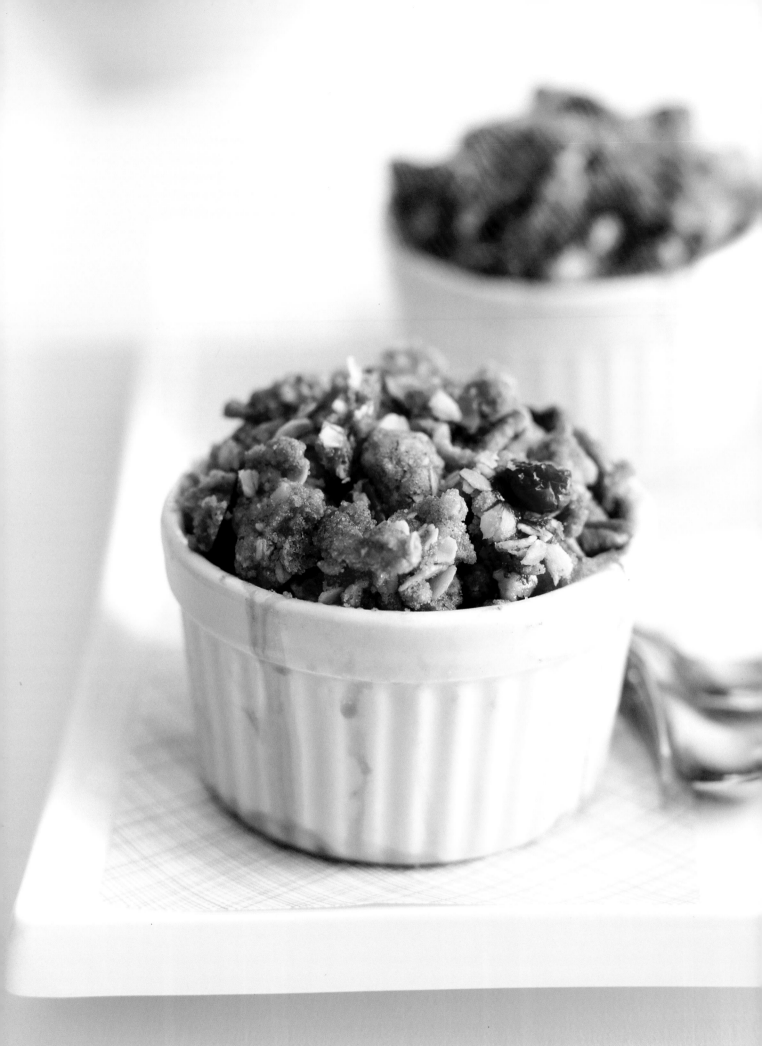

APPLE CRANBERRY CRISP

Makes one 8-inch (20 cm) square crisp or 6 individual crisps

The most comforting of fall desserts. And you can have a crisp in the oven within a matter of minutes.

FRESH TAKE

· This is such an easy recipe to remember that, after you've made it just once, or twice at the most, you'll have the proportions committed to memory.

· If I'm making just a straight apple crisp, without the tart cranberries, I don't bother with the added sugar.

Topping

½ cup	all-purpose flour	125 mL
½ cup	rolled oats	125 mL
½ cup	packed dark brown sugar	125 mL
5 Tbsp	unsalted butter, at room temperature	75 mL
1 tsp	ground cinnamon	5 mL
pinch	salt	pinch
½ cup	chopped pecans	125 mL

Fruit

4	Mutsu or Granny Smith apples, peeled, cored, and cut into ½-inch (1 cm) dice	4
1 cup	fresh or frozen cranberries	250 mL
⅓ cup	sugar	80 mL
	zest and juice of 1 small orange	

Preheat the oven to 325°F (160°C). Grease an 8-inch (20 cm) square baking dish or six 5 oz (150 mL) ramekins.

For the topping, combine the flour, oats, sugar, butter, cinnamon, and salt in a bowl. Work together with your fingertips until crumbly. Stir in the nuts and set aside.

For the fruit, toss the apples and cranberries with the sugar and orange zest and juice. Spoon it into the prepared baking dish(es) and sprinkle topping evenly overtop. Bake until bubbly and the apples are tender, about 30 minutes. Let cool slightly. Serve warm, topped with ice cream or cream, if desired.

Sweets

BAKED FIGS with HONEY & YOGURT *Serves 6*

You've got company coming, the roast is in the oven, and you suddenly realize you forgot about dessert! Never fear. You can have a simple, elegant dessert on the table in the blink of an eye.

FRESH TAKE

- Orange blossom water or rosewater, found at Middle Eastern or specialty food stores, is a nice added touch to the figs, but it's not essential. A dash of vanilla or almond extract will accomplish the same thing by adding a subtle yet complex taste.

- This is an ideal dessert for entertaining. It could be enjoyed with a glass of port or even the end of the red wine you might have served with the main course.

1 cup	full-fat yogurt	250 mL
3 + 6 Tbsp	honey	45 + 90 mL
1 Tbsp	finely chopped fresh mint	15 mL
dash	orange blossom water or rosewater	dash
12	fresh figs	12

Preheat the oven to 375°F (190°C).

Stir the yogurt with 3 Tbsp (45 mL) of the honey, the mint, and the flower water and chill until ready to serve.

Cut the figs in half, place them in a baking dish flat side up, and brush them with the remaining 6 Tbsp (90 mL) honey. Bake them for 10 minutes until warm.

Serve the figs warm with a spoonful of yogurt and a drizzle of honey.

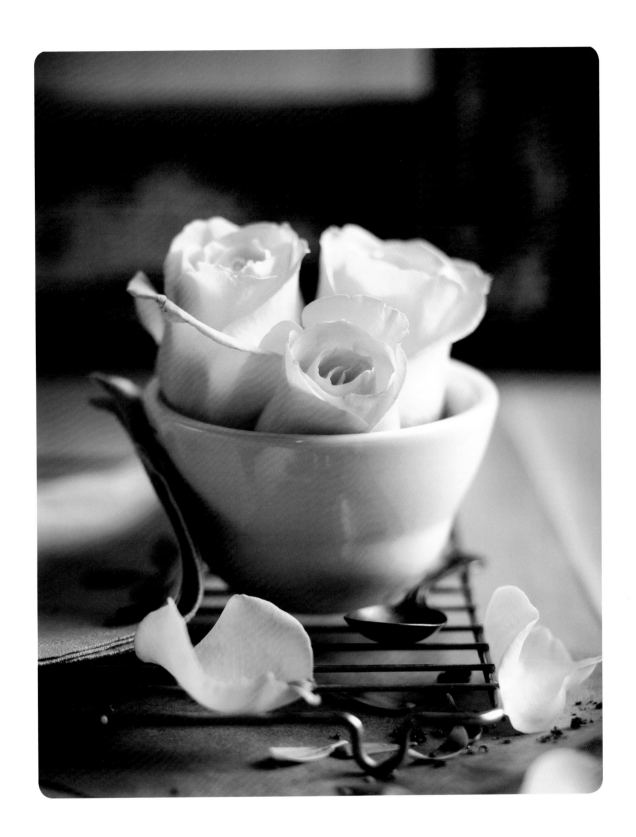

WINTER

As kids, we don't have a grasp of time or the future beyond "one more cartoon before bedtime" or "two more sleeps 'til Christmas," so the long grip of winter doesn't really mean anything until we grow up.

But because I love the change of seasons, I can't really gripe about winter. For me, it's the time to catch up on rest, to read, and to feel absolutely no guilt about spending a whole day indoors. My beagle, Oscar, curls up on the couch with me, ensuring that I can't go anywhere. I call it "couch yoga"—the reclined, stretched position reaching out for the remote control.

And the food of winter suits that attitude—slow-cooked meals, with heartiness built in. In winter we pay a premium for produce, so we counter that by braising more affordable cuts of meat. Comfort is the key, and while perhaps an overused term, still fits the bill.

And take heart . . . spring is just around the corner.

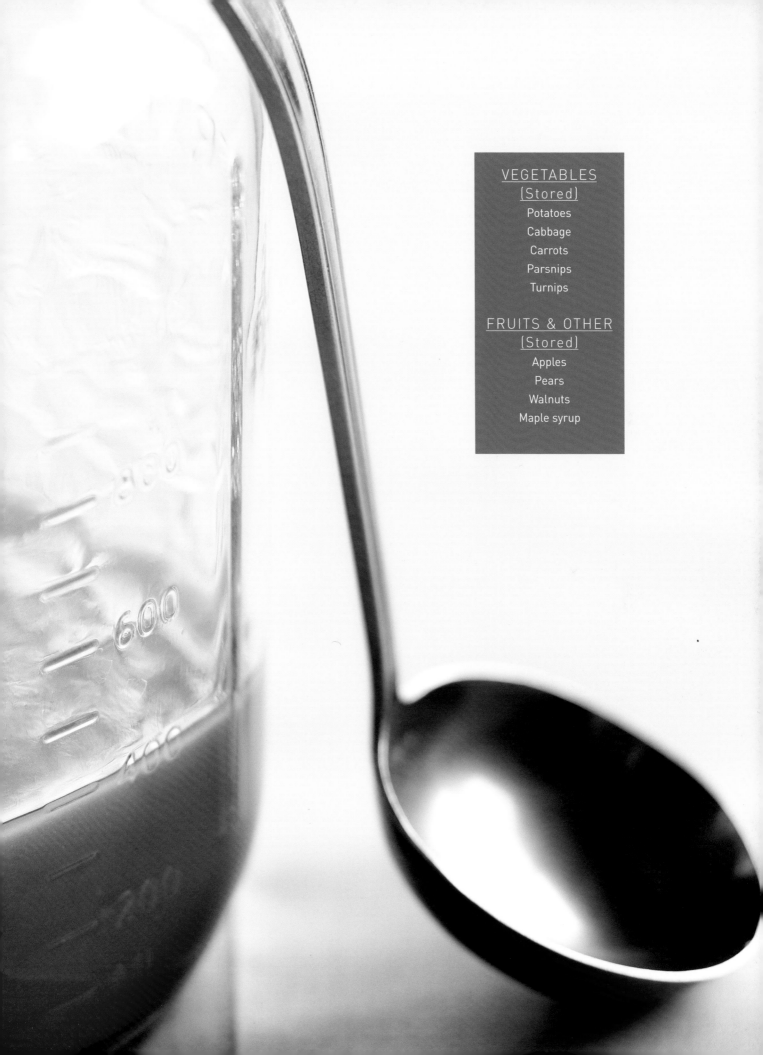

VEGETABLES
(Stored)
Potatoes
Cabbage
Carrots
Parsnips
Turnips

FRUITS & OTHER
(Stored)
Apples
Pears
Walnuts
Maple syrup

POTATO SOUP with BACON & CHEDDAR

Serves 6

A good potato soup can warm you even on the coldest day, especially when it's topped with bacon and cheddar, just like a baked potato.

FRESH TAKE

- A loaded baked potato is a beautiful thing, but this soup has a little more refinement to it. Straining the soup gives it a smooth, velvety texture, and the garnishes of bacon, cheddar, and chives aren't so overwhelming that they take over.

- Leeks are a natural companion to potatoes, especially in soup. Too often potato plays second fiddle to more dominant ingredients, but this soup is all about the taste and texture of that tuber. Leeks are milder than onions and give the soup depth without taking over.

- A little bit of cream, or in this case sour cream, helps to enrich a soup. For a dairy-free version simply replace the sour cream with the same measure of chicken stock.

4 strips	bacon, diced	4 strips
1½ cups	chopped leeks, white and light green parts only	375 mL
1½ lb	Yukon Gold potatoes, peeled and diced	750 g
5 cups	chicken stock	1.25 L
1 Tbsp	chopped fresh thyme	15 mL
1 cup	full-fat sour cream	250 mL
	salt & pepper	
1 cup	grated old cheddar	250 mL
2 Tbsp	chopped fresh chives or finely chopped green onion, for serving	30 mL

In a large pot, cook the bacon over medium heat until crisp. Remove the bacon and set it aside. Reduce the heat to medium-low and cook the leeks in the bacon fat until soft, about 5 minutes. Add the potatoes, chicken stock, and thyme, cover the pot loosely, and simmer until the potatoes are tender, about 20 minutes. Remove from the heat and purée. Strain the soup through a sieve and return the pot to medium heat. Stir in the sour cream and season to taste.

Serve the bowls of soup garnished with grated cheddar, the reserved bacon, and a sprinkle of chives or green onion.

VEGETABLE CHOWDER *Serves 6*

Stocked with veggies, this is a soup that makes a meal. Serve with bread, cheese, and a side salad and everybody in your house will be happy.

FRESH TAKE

· Three elements define a chowder: bacon, potato, and milk. While this chowder counts as the "real deal," for a vegetarian chowder you can skip the bacon (just sauté the vegetables in 2 Tbsp/ 30 mL olive oil) and use vegetable stock instead of chicken stock.

· The ratio of vegetables to liquid is almost two to one, which is why this is more of a meal, like a vegetable stew, than a regular soup.

· Thyme, oregano, and bay leaf are indispensable winter herbs. They work in just about every stew, and they are hardy enough to last in your garden or in your fridge unlike fragile basil or cilantro.

4 strips	bacon, diced	4 strips
1 cup	diced onion	250 mL
½ cup	diced celery	125 mL
½ cup	diced carrot	125 mL
1 cup	diced zucchini	250 mL
1 cup	broccoli florets	250 mL
1 cup	cauliflower florets	250 mL
½ cup	diced red bell pepper	125 mL
2 Tbsp	unsalted butter	30 mL
3 Tbsp	all-purpose flour	45 mL
2 cups	chicken stock	500 mL
2 cups	2% milk	500 mL
1 cup	fresh or frozen corn kernels	250 mL
1 cup	peeled and diced Yukon Gold potato	250 mL
2 tsp	chopped fresh thyme	10 mL
2 tsp	chopped fresh oregano	10 mL
1	bay leaf	1
	salt & pepper	

In a medium saucepot, cook the bacon over medium heat until crispy. Remove the bacon from the pan, leaving the fat, and set aside. Add the onion, celery, and carrot and sauté until translucent, about 5 minutes. Add the zucchini, broccoli, cauliflower, and red bell pepper and sauté for another 3 minutes. Remove the vegetables from the pot and set aside.

Melt the butter and add the flour to the pot. Stir constantly until you notice a nutty aroma, about 5 minutes. With a whisk, stir in the chicken stock a little at a time. Whisk in the milk in a slow stream. Return the vegetables to the pot, add the corn, potatoes, thyme, oregano, and bay leaf, and bring everything up to a simmer. Cover the pot and simmer the soup until the potatoes are tender, about 20 minutes. Add the reserved bacon and season to taste. Remove the bay leaf before serving.

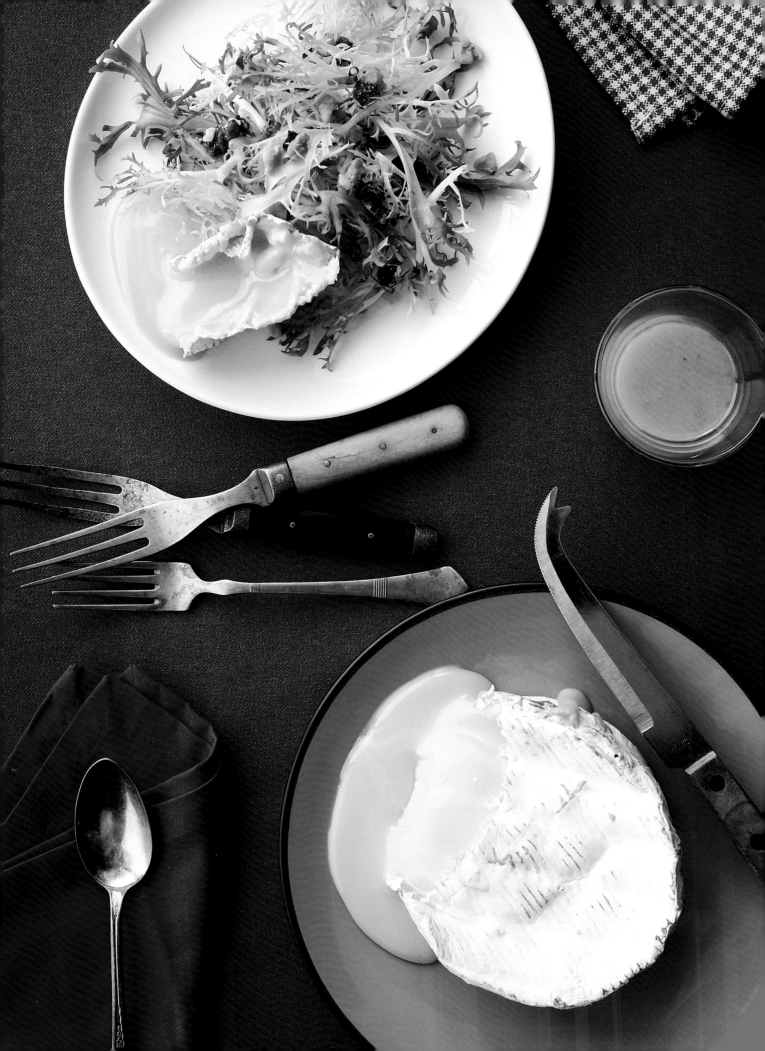

FRISÉE SALAD with WARM CAMEMBERT

Serves 4

Why save warm Camembert for an appetizer, covered in cranberry sauce or tapenade? Spoon it onto a salad, served after a main course for a cheese–meets–salad course.

FRESH TAKE

- Frisée is a feathery, light-colored lettuce with only a mild bitterness to it, unlike other bitter greens like radicchio or escarole. Be sure to buy mostly light green or yellow frisée for the mildest taste.

- My inspiration for this salad is the French *salade au lardons*, a frisée salad topped with cooked bacon and a poached egg. When you break into the egg, it coats the lettuce like a creamy dressing. I find the warm Camembert does the same thing here.

- It can be challenging to tell the ripeness of a brie or Camembert when it's a whole wheel. Gently press the center of the wheel. If it "gives" when gently pressed, then it's ripe, but if it still feels firm give it a week to ripen in the fridge. Baking the cheese does turn the center fluid, but an under-ripe cheese will still have a solid, chalky core to it.

Salad

1–2 heads	frisée lettuce	1–2 heads
1	green onion, chopped	1
½ cup	walnut pieces, lightly toasted	125 mL
7 oz	Camembert or brie cheese (whole, small wheel)	200 g

Vinaigrette (makes enough for many salads)

¼ cup	red wine vinegar	60 mL
1 tsp	Dijon mustard	5 mL
1 tsp	honey or sugar	5 mL
1 clove	garlic, minced	1 clove
	fine sea salt and ground black pepper	
¾ cup	extra virgin olive oil	185 mL

For the salad, cut the bottoms off the frisée leaves, then wash the leaves and arrange them on a platter. Sprinkle with chopped green onion and walnut pieces.

For the vinaigrette, whisk the red wine vinegar with the Dijon mustard, honey or sugar, garlic, and salt and pepper to taste until fully blended. Slowly pour in the oil, whisking constantly. The vinaigrette can be prepared in advance. Simply whisk it to emulsify it before drizzling over the salad.

Preheat the oven to 375°F (190°C).

Place the whole cheese on a baking tray and bake it for 12 minutes. Place it on the table next to the salad so that everyone can spoon out as much as they want.

CHORIZO CHEESE POTATO WRAPS

Makes 12 wraps • Serves 4

I've called these "wraps" because the potato slices wrap or cover chorizo and cheese inside, making a tasty and portable snack.

FRESH TAKE

· Weighing down the "wraps" with a baking tray keeps them compressed and flat, and also helps to crisp them up. They're really like a potato chip filled with cheese and sausage. Hungry yet?

· To really keep things Spanish, use grated manchego cheese in place of the cheddar.

· I designed this snack as something I could bring to a fall charity golf tournament. I rode around the course in a cart and handed out these potato treats to the golfers while they played. I seem to end up at the driving range every spring, and vow that in the summer I *will* become a golfer. This is the year, I can feel it!

	vegetable oil, for brushing	
3	large russet potatoes	3
12 thin slices	cured chorizo sausage (or cooked)	12 thin slices
1 cup	grated old cheddar cheese	250 mL

Preheat the oven to 400°F (200°C). Line a baking tray with parchment paper and brush the parchment with oil.

Peel the potatoes and slice them lengthwise into 24 slices, just under ¼ inch (6 mm) thick (using a mandolin is easiest). Place 12 potato slices on the prepared baking tray. Arrange a slice of chorizo on each potato slice and sprinkle with cheese, leaving the edges of the potato clear. Cover the cheese with the remaining potato slices. Place a sheet of parchment paper over the "wraps" and place a second baking tray on top. Bake for 15 minutes, then remove the top baking tray and parchment paper and bake until the potatoes are golden brown, about 8 minutes more.

Serve the "wraps" warm or at room temperature.

WALNUT BRIE STRUDEL

Makes three 16-inch (40 cm) strudels (about 36 bite-sized portions)

Strudel isn't just for apples! This stretched dough can envelop any sort of filling, but brie and walnuts with a hint of garlic win the prize here.

FRESH TAKE

- This is an authentic pulled strudel dough. Don't panic if the dough keeps springing back on you when you're stretching it—just take a break. The key to success is patience. Cover the dough with a tea towel and let it sit for five minutes before you resume stretching it—you'll find it will release its tension (as will you!) and go with the flow.

- These are hors d'oeuvre—sized strudels so you don't have to use a large tablecloth and stretch the dough five feet across. You'll find two feet is enough to roll up the filling and make many flaky layers.

- Brushing the dough with butter and sprinkling it with breadcrumbs is critical. The butter and breadcrumbs keep the layers separate once they've been rolled, so the dough remains separate and flaky.

Dough

1¼ cups	hot water	310 mL
⅓ cup	unsalted butter, melted	80 mL
4 cups	bread flour	1 L
½ cup + 2 Tbsp	sugar	125 mL + 30 mL
½ tsp	salt	2 mL

Filling

1 cup	creamy ricotta cheese	250 mL
1 clove	garlic, minced	1 clove
6 oz	brie	175 g
¼ tsp	black pepper	1 mL
3 cups	walnut pieces, lightly toasted	750 mL

Assembly

⅔ cup	unsalted butter, melted	160 mL
1½ cups	dry breadcrumbs	375 mL
1	egg mixed with 2 Tbsp (30 mL) water, for brushing	1
1½ Tbsp	poppyseeds	22.5 mL

For the dough, place all the dough ingredients in the bowl of an electric mixer fitted with the paddle attachment. Mix for 2 minutes on low speed, and then increase the speed to medium.

Knead the dough for 10 minutes, pulling it off the paddle once or twice, until it takes on a stringy appearance. Wrap the dough in plastic wrap and let it rest at room temperature for at least 1 hour before using and up to 3 hours. If chilling (you can make and chill this dough up to 2 days in advance), let the dough come fully to room temperature before the pulling process.

For the filling, stir together the ricotta and garlic. Cut the brie into small pieces and beat it vigorously into the ricotta. Stir in the pepper and chill until ready to assemble.

Continued . . .

Preheat the oven to 375°F (190°C). Line a baking tray with parchment paper.

Lay a small tablecloth over a work surface, with some of the tabletop showing, and sprinkle the cloth with flour. Cut the dough into 3 pieces. Coat your hands with flour and press flat the first piece of dough. Carefully start stretching the dough into a square shape, pulling gently and evenly. It's easiest if you use the back of your hands. The strudel dough should stretch to about 16 × 24 inches (40 × 60 cm), with the shorter end facing you. The dough should be very thin—as thin if not thinner than phyllo. Use the table or counter edge to secure the dough once it's almost the right size (these are small strudels, so they won't take up the whole table).

Brush the entire surface lightly with melted butter and sprinkle it with ½ cup (125 mL) breadcrumbs. Spoon one-third of the cheese filling about 1 inch (2.5 cm) thick along 1 side of the strudel. Sprinkle 1 cup (250 mL) of walnuts over the cheese filling and a little over the dough. Trim the edges of the strudel dough. Lift the dough up using the tablecloth from the cheese-filled end and let the pastry roll itself up as you lift the cloth. Pinch the ends closed and lift it onto the prepared tray. Brush the top with egg wash and sprinkle with poppyseeds. Repeat this with the remaining 2 pieces of dough.

Bake the strudels for 18 to 25 minutes, until rich golden brown. Cool for 15 minutes before slicing.

Serve this strudel on its own, as an appetizer with a salad, or as a starch for a main course.

ANTIPASTI

A few homemade accoutrements can take sliced meats and cheeses to a new level of spectacular.

FRESH TAKE

- Making marinated artichokes from fresh is really worth the effort. I find the buttery taste and texture of freshly cooked and dressed artichokes beats out the jarred version.

- The pickled mushrooms pack a punch, but as the balsamic vinegar reduces and absorbs into the mushrooms, there is a bit of sweetness produced that rounds out every morsel.

- Need to add olives to your antipasti platter? Toss kalamata olives with a little chopped rosemary, some black pepper, and a chopped green onion to make a trio of marinated delights.

MARINATED ARTICHOKE HEARTS
Makes about 2 cups (500 mL)

4	large artichokes (or 8 small)	4
2	lemons, plus a lemon half	2
2 Tbsp	extra virgin olive oil	30 mL
1 clove	garlic, minced	1 clove
2 Tbsp	chopped fresh oregano	30 mL
	salt & pepper	

Trim the tops off of the artichoke leaves and rub the cut portions with a lemon half. Place the artichokes in a pot and cover them with water. Squeeze in the juice of the 2 lemons and drop all the lemon halves into the water. Simmer the artichokes until their base pierces easily with a fork, about 40 minutes. Drain and cool.

To prepare the hearts, pull away the leaves and remove the spiny center of the heart. Peel the outside of the stem with a paring knife and cut the hearts into quarters. Toss the quarters with the remaining ingredients and season to taste. Chill until ready to serve.

QUICK PICKLED MUSHROOMS
Makes about 3 cups (750 mL)

2 Tbsp	olive oil	30 mL
1½ lb	fresh button or cremini mushrooms, kept whole but with stems trimmed	750 g
½ cup	balsamic vinegar	125 mL
1 clove	garlic, minced	1 clove
1 tsp	chopped fresh thyme	5 mL
	salt & pepper	

In a sauté pan over medium-high heat, add the oil and whole mushrooms. Sauté until all the liquid from the mushrooms evaporates, about 5 minutes. Add the vinegar, garlic, and thyme and continue to cook until the balsamic is absorbed, about 3 minutes. Remove from the heat, cool to room temperature, then season to taste.

Store the mushrooms refrigerated, but serve them at room temperature.

PAN-ROASTED TROUT with LEEKS & BROWN BUTTER *Serves 6*

Fresh trout is beautifully mild and flaky. By serving it with a classic brown butter sauce and croutons to soak up all the juices, its lean character and mild taste is accentuated.

FRESH TAKE

- Trout fillets are typically sold with the pin bones removed, but it's a good idea to double check. Run a finger across the center of the fillet, back and forth—you'll feel any bones that are left. A pair of tweezers is the best way to extract them.

- Trout is typically cooked with its skin on. It's so tender that a skinless fillet would shatter into flaky shards the moment you tried to lift it.

- I learned to cook this dish when I worked in New Orleans, but my finest memory is having it prepared by charismatic Chef Bourassa at Café Henri Burger in Hull, Quebec. Michael and I were guest chefs in his kitchen, and he had just caught the fish fly-fishing that morning. We truly ate at the chef's table that afternoon!

Clarified Butter

1 cup	unsalted butter	250 mL

Croutons

1½ cups	French bread, cut into ½-inch (1 cm) cubes	375 mL
3 Tbsp	melted clarified butter	45 mL
1 clove	garlic, minced	1 clove
2 Tbsp	finely chopped flat-leaf parsley	30 mL
	salt & pepper	

Trout

7 Tbsp	melted clarified butter, divided, for the leeks and the fish; remaining clarified butter to go in the sauce	105 mL
¾ cup	chopped leeks, white and light green parts only	185 mL
½ tsp	chopped fresh thyme	2 mL
	salt & pepper	
6	trout fillets (about 6 oz/175 g each), pin bones removed	6
2	lemons	2
½ cup	coarsely chopped flat-leaf parsley	125 mL

For the clarified butter, heat the butter in a small pot over medium-low heat until melted. Remove the pot from the heat and let it sit for 5 minutes. Slowly and carefully pour or ladle out the butter into a bowl, until you reach the milky solids (which can be discarded). Use the butter now or chill it for later use.

Preheat the oven to 350°F (180°C). Line a baking pan with parchment paper.

For the croutons, toss the bread with the 3 Tbsp (45 mL) butter and the garlic and parsley and season. Spread the bread onto the prepared baking tray and toast it for 12 to 18 minutes, stirring once or twice, until golden brown. Cool the croutons and store them in a resealable container until ready to use.

Continued . . .

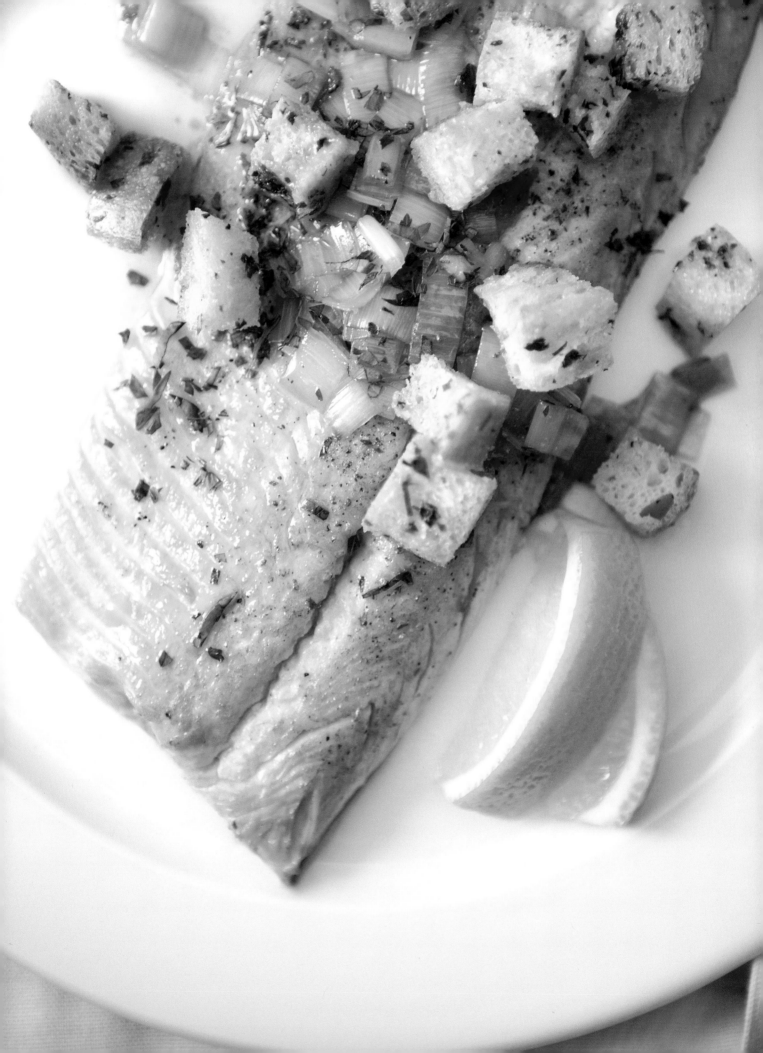

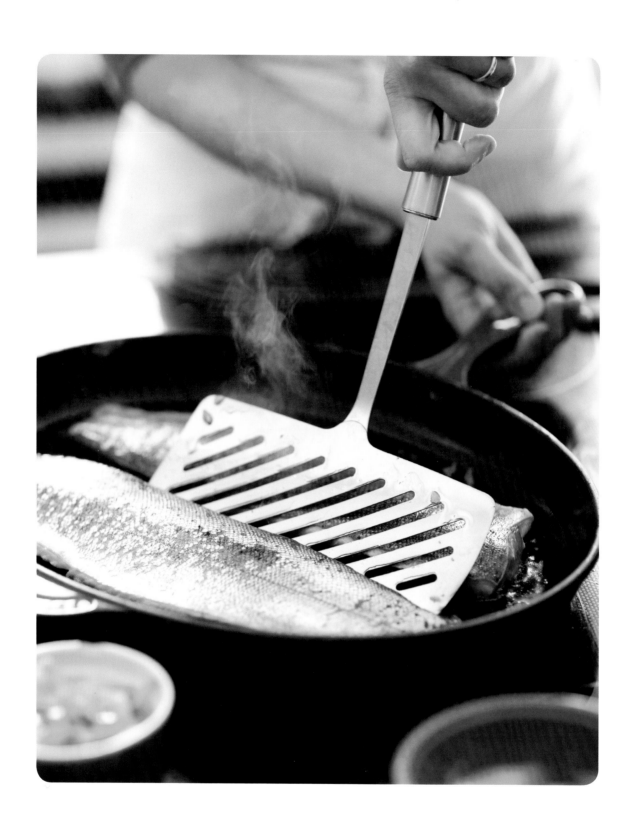

For the trout, keep the oven temperature at 350°F (180°C) and line another baking pan with parchment paper.

Heat a large sauté pan over medium heat and add 1 Tbsp (15 mL) of the melted clarified butter. Add the leeks and thyme and cook, stirring often, until the leeks are tender, about 5 minutes. Season lightly and remove from the pan. Increase the heat to medium-high and add 2 Tbsp (30 mL) clarified butter. Season the trout lightly and place 2 fillets, skin side up, in the pan. Cook for 4 minutes, until the fish have browned, then gently transfer them to the prepared baking pan, skin side down. Add another 2 Tbsp (30 mL) of the butter and repeat with 2 more fillets, then repeat the whole process with the last 2 fillets. (Set aside the sauté pan.) Bake for about 10 minutes, until the fish yields when touched with a fork.

To finish the sauce, cook the remaining butter in the same sauté pan over medium heat until browned. Add the leeks to warm them through. Add the juice of 1 lemon, parsley, and salt and pepper to taste. Stir in the croutons immediately before serving.

To serve, place the trout on a plate or platter, and top with the croutons and the leeks. Serve immediately.

MAPLE-ROASTED CHICKEN BREASTS *Serves 8*

If you like honey garlic chicken wings, you'll love these baked (not fried!) chicken breasts.

FRESH TAKE

- B-grade maple syrup is a darker, slightly stronger-tasting syrup, used for cooking because of its full body. If B-grade isn't available, marinate the chicken in 1 cup (250 mL) of A-grade, but for the sauce, use ⅔ cup (160 mL) of A-grade and simmer for 10 minutes (instead of 3) to reduce it and concentrate the taste.

- These chicken breasts make a great club sandwich if you have any leftovers. I think it's the maple syrup on the chicken that goes well with bacon on a club—you know how tasty it is when maple syrup from your pancakes spills onto your bacon at breakfast!

- This is real comfort food. The house smells great as the chicken cooks, and if you serve this with the Three-Cheese Pasta Bake (page 161) you'll send your family over the top with joy.

8	boneless, skinless chicken breasts	8
1½ cups	B-grade pure maple syrup, divided	375 mL
1 head	garlic	1 head
⅓ cup + 3 Tbsp	malt vinegar	80 mL + 45 mL
	salt & pepper	

Place the chicken breasts in a shallow dish. Pour 1 cup (250 mL) of the maple syrup overtop. Peel all the garlic cloves, crush them under the flat side of a knife, and add all but 2 cloves to the chicken. Add ⅓ cup (80 mL) of the malt vinegar, toss the chicken to coat, and marinate for 1 to 6 hours.

Preheat the oven to 375°F (190°C). Grease a roasting pan.

Place the chicken breasts in the roasting pan, shaking off any excess syrup, and season. Roast, uncovered, for about 25 minutes, until an internal temperature of 180°F (82°C) is reached. Let the chicken rest 10 minutes.

To serve, heat the remaining ½ cup (125 mL) maple syrup, 3 Tbsp (45 mL) malt vinegar, and 2 cloves of garlic. Simmer for 3 minutes, remove the garlic, and keep the syrup warm. Slice the chicken breasts into 3 pieces on an angle and plate. Spoon warm syrup over and serve.

ROSEMARY ROASTED LAMB with
DATE PISTACHIO "SALSA" *Serves 6*

A special occasion warrants a special cut of meat, and lamb rack is a deserving choice. Instead of a reduction or heavy sauce, I've opted for a colorful "salsa" that pairs beautifully with the rich lamb. This dish is worthy of a decadent wine selection.

FRESH TAKE

- Lamb racks are usually sold frenched, meaning the ends of the rib bones have been cleaned of excess trim and fat. It's an elegant presentation and makes the racks easy to handle for slicing.

- Medjool dates originally hail from Morocco, and are usually sold with their pits intact, but the pits are easily removed by slicing the dates open before chopping. Medjool dates are quite moist for a dried fruit, but they'll still absorb the red wine sprinkled over them for the salsa.

- A rich red wine like a Cabernet Sauvignon, Shiraz, or Zinfandel works well with this dish. If you're making the salsa an hour or so before dinner guests arrive, you can open a bottle and use it in the salsa. Since the salsa is not cooked, the full profile of the wine will show through.

Lamb

2 tsp	cumin seed	10 mL
2 tsp	coriander seed	10 mL
1½ tsp	salt	7.5 mL
1 tsp	ground black pepper	5 mL
1 tsp	dry mustard	5 mL
3 Tbsp	chopped fresh rosemary	45 mL
3 Tbsp	olive oil	45 mL
3	lamb racks, frenched	3

"Salsa"

1 cup	pitted and chopped Medjool dates	250 mL
⅓ cup	finely diced red onion	80 mL
2 Tbsp	red wine	30 mL
½ cup	chopped pistachios	125 mL
3 oz	fresh goat cheese	90 g

For the lamb, toast the cumin and coriander in a sauté pan, tossing, until the fragrance becomes rich, about 2 minutes. In a mortar and pestle or in a small food processor, grind all the spices with the rosemary and olive oil to create a paste.

Preheat the oven to 375°F (190°C).

Cut the lamb racks in half, rub their surface with the paste, and place them in a roasting pan. Roast for about 18 minutes for medium doneness (an internal temperature of 135°F/57°C). Let the lamb rest for 10 minutes before slicing and plating.

For the "salsa," toss the dates and red onion with the wine and let them sit for 5 minutes to soften. Stir in the pistachios and serve with the lamb, crumbling goat cheese on top.

Meat

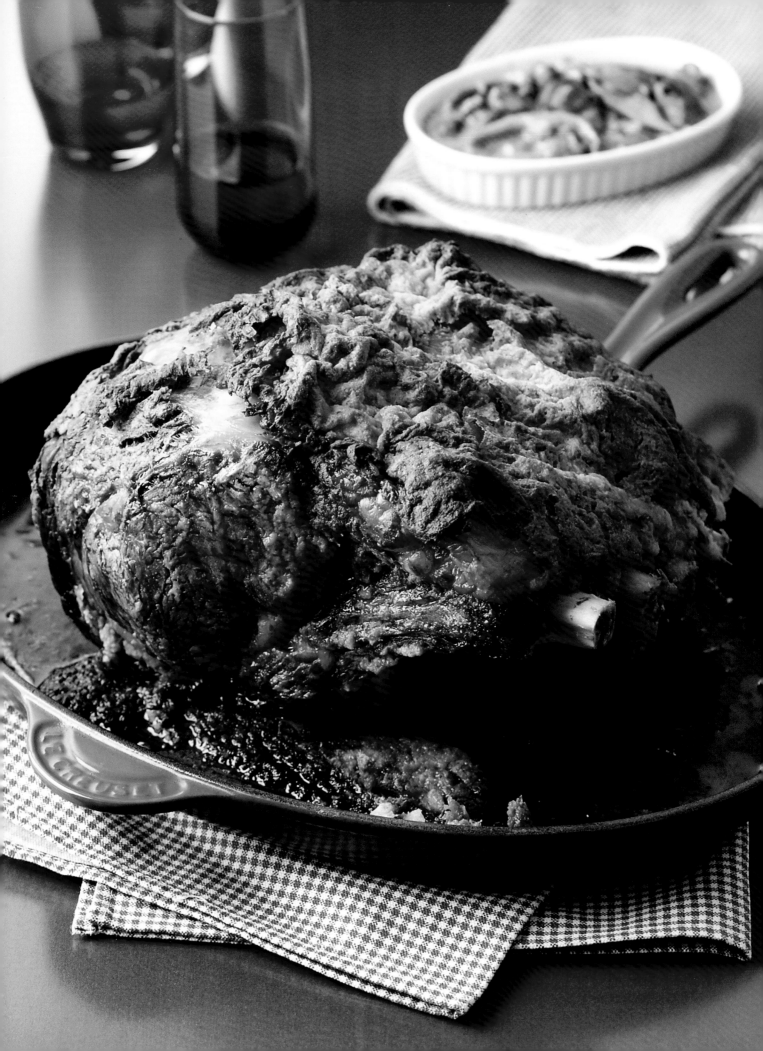

SLOW-ROASTED PRIME RIB with MUSHROOM JUS *Serves 8*

The Rolls Royce of roast beef. Slow-roasting it is the most loving way to treat such a tasty cut.

FRESH TAKE

- Mushrooms and beef are a natural pairing. Chanterelles are a rich-tasting, tender, orange-brown mushroom that you can find at specialty food stores. If they're not available, use other wild mushrooms or cremini mushrooms in their place.

- Slow-roasting is wise for such a large roast. It ensures the heat gradually and evenly permeates the meat so that a medium-rare roast is an even pink color all the way through, and not well done on the outside with just a pink center. Investing in a good digital probe thermometer is also a wise idea.

- Oh goodness, I go weak at the knees when I pull this roast from the oven. The mustard and horseradish salt crust becomes a crispy coating, just daring me to pull off a piece and crunch on it. Maybe just a little bit—no one will notice.

½	whole prime rib roast, about 8 lb (3.5 kg)	½
½ cup	Dijon mustard	125 mL
⅓ cup	prepared horseradish	80 mL
3 Tbsp	salt	45 mL
2 Tbsp	ground black pepper	30 mL

Preheat the oven to 325°F (160°C).

Place the roast upright in a roasting pan. Stir together the mustard, horseradish, salt, and pepper and rub over the surface of the roast. Place uncovered on the oven's center rack and cook for 2 to 2½ hours, to an internal temperature of 130°F (54°C) for rare. Transfer to a cutting board and rest, tented with tinfoil, for at least 15 minutes before carving. Use a sharp knife to carefully slice down and remove the bones. Carve thin or thick slices of beef, as desired.

MUSHROOM JUS
Makes about 3 cups (750 mL)

2	shallots, sliced	2
2 cups	chanterelles, or other mushrooms such as cremini, oyster, and/or shiitake	500 mL
2 Tbsp	all-purpose flour	30 mL
2 cups	chicken or beef stock	500 mL
2 tsp	chopped fresh thyme	10 mL
¼ cup	brandy	60 mL
⅓ cup	whipping cream	80 mL
	coarse salt and ground black pepper	

Take the roasting pan from the prime rib roast and drain off all but 2 Tbsp (30 mL) of the drippings. Over medium heat, sauté the shallots and mushrooms in the drippings until soft, about 8 minutes. Add the flour and cook over medium heat for 3 minutes, until the flour is worked into a paste. Add the stock gradually (whisking it in slowly to avoid lumps), stir in the thyme, and bring to a full simmer. Add the brandy, simmer for 2 minutes more, then add the cream. Return to a simmer then season to taste and serve.

Meat

BRAISED BEEF SHORT RIBS *Serves 4*

Well-made short ribs make your lips stick together when you eat them. Make sure you have lots of bread handy to soak up all those tasty juices.

FRESH TAKE

- Braisable cuts like short ribs have a lot going for them. Because there are more short ribs than, say, tenderloins (consider—there are only two tenderloins on a beef steer), they're affordable. And because these cuts are typically well exercised, they have fantastically rich flavor. The toughness that comes with that? Well, the slow, moist cooking process takes care of that!

- I like to dredge (or coat) my short ribs with cornstarch instead of flour. I find that flour tends to scorch in the pot when searing, or sinks to the bottom and sticks once the liquid is added. Cornstarch doesn't do this, but it does thicken the sauce as it cooks, which is what you want.

- Adding juniper, balsamic, and figs is my little "tart-up" for what is essentially simple, humble food. These additions really add great character and balance the richness of the beef itself.

4 pieces	bone-in beef short ribs (about 8 oz/250 g each)	4 pieces
2 Tbsp	cornstarch	30 mL
1 Tbsp	olive oil	15 mL
4	medium carrots, peeled and diced (½-inch/1 cm dice)	4
1	medium onion, peeled and diced (½-inch/1 cm dice)	1
4 cloves	garlic, minced	4 cloves
1	28 oz (796 mL) can diced tomatoes	1
1 cup	dry red wine	250 mL
4 cups	chicken stock	1 L
2 sprigs	fresh thyme	2 sprigs
2	bay leaves	2
1 Tbsp	juniper berries	15 mL
2 Tbsp	balsamic vinegar	30 mL
6	dried figs, finely chopped	6
	salt & pepper	

Preheat the oven to 300°F (150°C).

Pat the beef dry and dredge it in the cornstarch, shaking off any excess. Heat the oil over medium-high heat in a heavy-bottomed pot, brown the beef on all sides, and set aside. Reduce the heat to medium and sauté the carrots and onion until the onion is translucent, about 5 minutes. Add the garlic and sauté for 1 minute more. Add the tomatoes, wine, stock, thyme, bay leaves, and juniper berries and return to a simmer. Return the beef to the pot, cover, and transfer to the oven. Cook the short ribs for 2 hours, then add the vinegar. Cook for another 2 hours, until the flesh pulls away easily from the bone. Skim off any excess fat from the surface. Before serving, stir in the figs and season to taste.

Meat

ISRAELI COUSCOUS with
OLIVES, ARUGULA, & FETA *Serves 8*

In the middle of winter, you sometimes need a break from potato dishes or other heavy-duty carbs. This couscous has hints of summer vibrance, but it's a tasty side for a braised dish like a lamb stew or even Osso Buco (page 110).

FRESH TAKE

- Israeli couscous is, like regular couscous, basically a pasta as it's made from rolled durum wheat. Israeli couscous has larger grains than regular couscous, though, and it cooks up to the size of tapioca pearls. If you can't find it, simply use traditional couscous.

- I included this recipe because in midwinter, all these ingredients are both available and tasty.

1 cup	Israeli couscous	250 mL
2 Tbsp	extra virgin olive oil	30 mL
1 bunch	arugula, washed and coarsely chopped	1 bunch
1 cup	pitted and chopped kalamata or taggiasca olives	250 mL
½ cup	minced red onion	125 mL
½ cup	crumbled feta cheese	125 mL
¼ cup	minced celery	60 mL
1 Tbsp	lemon juice	15 mL
	salt & pepper	

Bring 1¼ cups (310 mL) lightly salted water up to a boil. Add the couscous, stir, and reduce the heat to medium. Cook, uncovered, stirring occasionally, until all the liquid has been absorbed. Scrape the couscous into a strainer and rinse it under cold water to cool. Transfer the couscous to a bowl and toss with the olive oil to coat. Add the arugula, olives, onion, feta, celery, and lemon juice and toss. Season to taste and chill until ready to serve.

The couscous can be prepared up to 8 hours in advance.

Starch

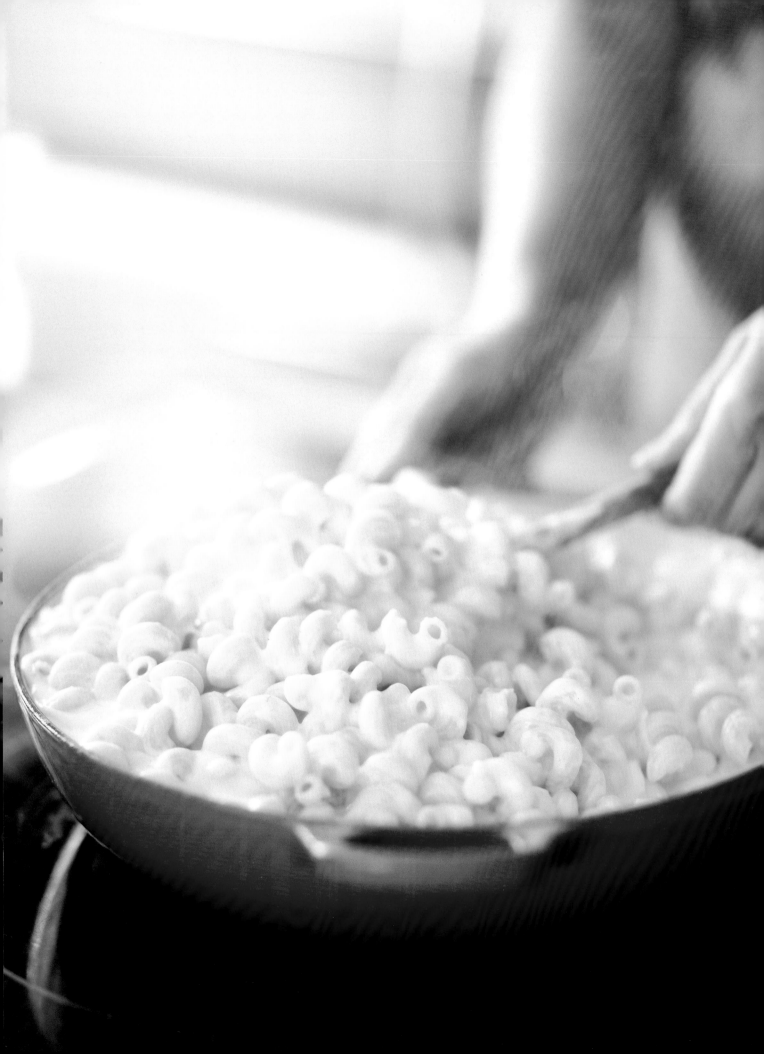

THREE-CHEESE PASTA BAKE *Serves 8*

Ah yes, macaroni and cheese. This dish is probably number two on the top ten list of comfort food, second only to mashed potatoes. It's wonderful with Maple-Roasted Chicken Breasts (page 154).

(page 154).

FRESH TAKE

· Making a good cheese sauce is rooted in the world of classic French sauce preparation. This recipe is a textbook Mornay sauce. The end result might be humble and comforting, but the technique is 100 percent professional.

· Cream cheese is my little trick here (as in the quesadillas too, page 145). It keeps the sauce smooth, and its "tang" keeps the sauce from tasting too heavy.

· I don't rinse pasta if it's to be served immediately, but here, rinsing halts the cooking—I find that freshly cooked pasta baked with a warm sauce will keep cooking and get mushy. Rinsing also removes the surface starch ensuring that the pasta won't soak up too much of the sauce it's baked in.

· There's no technical chef's secret behind cooling the dish for 10 minutes before serving. If you take a bite of the bubbling cheesy goodness without waiting first . . . ow!!!

1 lb	macaroni, or other small pasta	500 g
½ cup	unsalted butter	125 mL
½ cup	all-purpose flour	125 mL
4 cups	2% milk	1 L
⅛ tsp	ground nutmeg	0.5 mL
1	8 oz (225 g) pkg full-fat cream cheese	1
1½ cups	grated old cheddar cheese	375 mL
1 cup	grated Swiss Gruyère	250 mL
½ cup	dry breadcrumbs	125 mL

Bring a large pot of salted water to a boil. Add the macaroni and boil, uncovered, until just tender to taste. Drain, rinse with cold water, and set aside.

Preheat the oven to 350°F (180°C).

In a large pot, melt the butter over medium heat and add the flour. Stir this roux with a wooden or nonreactive spoon until it has a lightly nutty aroma but no color, about 5 minutes. Slowly whisk in the milk, then bring the entire mixture up to a simmer, whisking constantly. If you get lumps, strain the sauce and return it to the heat. Add the nutmeg and whisk in the cream cheese until smooth.

Reduce the heat to medium-low and stir in the cheddar and Gruyère until melted. Stir in the reserved macaroni and spoon into an 8-cup (2 L) baking dish. Sprinkle with the breadcrumbs and bake for 25 to 30 minutes, until bubbling around the edges.

Cool for 10 minutes before serving.

Starch

WINTER POTATO BEET SALAD *Serves 6*

A chilled potato salad does have a place on a cool-weather supper table, believe it or not. This is a fabulous dish to place on a buffet table next to a roasted ham. And it's perfect for a holiday open house.

FRESH TAKE

- I have to give full credit for this recipe to Ingrid Wilkins. She was our neighbor when I was growing up, and it was a tradition to go to her family's for dinner on Boxing Day. This salad was always on the table and I always looked forward to it. She and my mom still keep in touch, and she was kind enough to share the recipe.

- Cooked celery root has such a mild and pleasant creaminess to it. It completely melds with the other ingredients, and this and the beets make this recipe very different from a traditional summery potato salad.

1½ lb	Yukon Gold potatoes	750 g
1 lb	whole beets (about 4 medium)	500 g
1 lb	celery root (1 medium)	500 g
6 Tbsp	olive oil, divided	90 mL
	salt & pepper	
⅓ cup	full-fat sour cream	80 mL
¼ cup	mayonnaise	60 mL
1 Tbsp	white vinegar	15 mL
1 Tbsp	prepared horseradish	15 mL
1 tsp	Dijon mustard	5 mL
2 Tbsp	chopped fresh dill	30 mL

Preheat the oven to 350°F (180°C).

Peel and dice the potatoes, beets, and celery root. Place each vegetable in separate baking dishes, toss each with 2 Tbsp (30 mL) of the oil, and season lightly. Cover each dish with tinfoil and bake until tender. The celery root takes about 30 minutes, potatoes about 40 minutes, and beets, 50 minutes. Let cool.

Whisk together the sour cream, mayonnaise, vinegar, horseradish, mustard, and dill. Stir in the cooled vegetables and season to taste.

This salad is best prepared a day ahead and stirred a couple of times while it's chilling. The rosy beet color will permeate the salad.

BRAISED RED CABBAGE *Serves 10*

Properly cooked red cabbage is a beautiful thing, and very affordable, too!

FRESH TAKE

- Acidity, in the form of red wine vinegar, is essential to keep the red cabbage color bright. Without it the cabbage will turn a purplish blue and also taste rather flat.

- I like having the apple here—it softens and rounds out the taste of the whole dish. If you're a caraway fan, feel free to add a sprinkle.

- Michael laughs at me because it's in my nature to serve sour cream with cabbage, even here. If you haven't tried it, you should. It's like adding the dollop of sour cream to a bowl of borscht—it's meant to be!

2 Tbsp	unsalted butter	30 mL
1 cup	diced onion	250 mL
1	coarsely grated apple	1
½ head	red cabbage, cored and sliced	½ head
½ cup	apple cider	125 mL
3 Tbsp	red wine vinegar	45 mL
3 Tbsp	sugar	45 mL
¼ tsp	ground nutmeg	1 mL
	salt & pepper	

Melt the butter in a heavy-bottomed saucepot and cook the onion until translucent. Add the apple, cabbage, apple cider, vinegar, sugar, and nutmeg and simmer, covered, for 15 minutes or until the cabbage is tender. Season to taste and serve.

Vegetables

GRILLED APPLES & FENNEL *Serves 6*

Even though the weather cools off, many of us grill all year round. Even wintry ingredients like fennel and apples hint at warmer weather when grilled just a little.

FRESH TAKE

- The cranberry vinaigrette is a tasty alternative to a gravy or sauce served over roasted chicken breasts or with a roasted pork loin.

- I opt for Cortland apples here, since they stay nice and white once sliced. McIntosh is my number two choice, but you may have to toss them with a little lemon juice to keep them bright.

Cranberry Vinaigrette

1 cup	fresh or frozen cranberries	250 mL
⅓ cup	sugar	80 mL
¼ cup	finely minced onion	60 mL
1 tsp	finely chopped fresh rosemary	5 mL
1 tsp	Dijon mustard	5 mL
5 Tbsp	vegetable oil (or extra virgin soya oil)	75 mL
	salt & pepper	

Apples and Fennel

2	Cortland apples (or McIntosh)	2
½ head	fennel	½ head
2 Tbsp	vegetable oil	30 mL
	Treviso radicchio	

For the cranberry vinaigrette, simmer the cranberries, sugar, onion, and rosemary with ½ cup (125 mL) water until the cranberries "pop," about 20 minutes. Remove the pot from the heat and cool to room temperature. Whisk in the Dijon mustard, then slowly whisk in oil. Season to taste.

Preheat the grill to high heat.

Core the apples, keeping the skin on, and cut them into ¼-inch (6 mm) slices. Cut the fennel into slices of the same thickness, leaving the core in, then toss the apples and fennel in the oil. Grill them until lightly charred on both sides, but still crunchy, about 4 minutes in total.

To serve, arrange some radicchio leaves on a platter and arrange the apples and fennel on top. Spoon over the cranberry vinaigrette and serve.

Vegetables

MUSHROOM & SMOKED CHEDDAR FRITTATA

Serves 6

Smoked cheddar sends this easy egg dish to new levels of enjoyment. It also makes it one of the best breakfast dishes to serve for dinner.

FRESH TAKE

- A frittata is the easiest egg dish in the world to make. With scrambled eggs, fried eggs, and omelets, you have to work hard to avoid a crust on the eggs, but in a frittata you want that crust so the dish is easy to lift out, slice, and serve.

- Compared to button mushrooms, creminis have a firmer texture when cooked. They are great in a frittata, a nice "meaty" option if you want to keep it vegetarian.

- With a simple preparation like this, a humble ingredient like parsley plays an important role, bringing all the other flavors together. In a more complicated dish, the parsley would be lost, but here it holds its own.

8	eggs	8
¼ cup	olive oil	60 mL
1 lb	cremini mushrooms, sliced	500 g
1	clove garlic, minced	1
2 Tbsp	chopped flat-leaf parsley	30 mL
	salt & pepper	
1½ cups	coarsely grated smoked cheddar cheese	375 mL

Preheat the oven to 375°F (190°C).

Whisk the eggs with 2 Tbsp (30 mL) water and set aside. In a large ovenproof sauté pan over medium-high heat, add the olive oil. Add the mushrooms and sauté until tender and all the liquid has evaporated, about 5 minutes. Add the garlic and parsley and cook for 1 minute more. Stir in the parsley and season to taste. Pour the eggs over the mushrooms, stir to just combine them, then sprinkle over the grated cheese. Place the pan in the oven and bake, uncovered, until the eggs have set and the cheese has melted, about 15 minutes. Turn the frittata out onto a plate and cut it into wedges to serve.

MAPLE-BAKED APPLE BITES *Makes about 2 dozen bites*

Chips for breakfast? When they're crispy apple chips, with a little sprinkle of cinnamon and pecans on top, it's an innovative way to get the kids to eat their fruit.

FRESH TAKE

· The icing sugar and maple syrup turn into a candy and crisp up the apples slices as they dry and bake, and the sprinkling of pecans make them taste almost like a fruit crisp.

· Store these baked nibbles in an airtight container at room temperature for up to one week. If refrigerated, they'll go soft in just a few hours.

· What a perfect packed lunch treat for the kids! The apple bites can replace a cookie when you need to pack something sweet, and they transport very well—not too fragile at all.

6 Tbsp	icing sugar, divided	90 mL
6 Tbsp	pure maple syrup, divided	90 mL
2	Mutsu or Granny Smith apples	2
½ cup	finely chopped pecans	125 mL
pinch	ground cinnamon	pinch

Preheat the oven to 225°F (105°C). Line 2 large baking trays with parchment paper.

Whisk 3 Tbsp (45 mL) of the icing sugar with 3 Tbsp (45 mL) of the maple syrup and set aside. Sift the remaining 3 Tbsp (45 mL) icing sugar evenly onto the prepared baking trays. Using a mandolin or other manual slicer, cut the apples crosswise into paper-thin slices. (The apples do not need to be cored.) Arrange the apple slices in 1 layer on the prepared sheets and brush with the maple syrup mixture. Bake the slices for about 2 hours (rotating the pans halfway through cooking), or until they're pale golden and starting to crisp. Brush the cooked apple slices with the remaining 3 Tbsp (45 mL) maple syrup, sprinkle with chopped pecans and cinnamon, and bake for an additional 20 minutes. Immediately peel the apple bites off the parchment and cool on a rack.

PEANUT-BUTTER-&-JAM BREAD PUDDING

Makes one 9-inch (23 cm) square pan • Serves 8

I have a real weakness for a good peanut-butter-and-jam sandwich, and in dessert form it is just as comforting.

FRESH TAKE

- I prefer to use jam rather than a jelly in the bread pudding. Jam holds its own, and lightly cooked preserves with lots of fruit pieces are ideal.

- You can use crunchy or creamy peanut butter here. For a peanut-free version, melt the same measure of cream cheese in place of the peanut butter. (I like cream cheese and jam sandwiches, too.)

- This is one of those desserts that I like to serve just to have leftovers. A heaping spoonful of this, slightly warmed and enjoyed with a glass of cold milk, is my idea of a perfect bedtime snack.

¼ cup	unsalted butter	60 mL
⅔ cup	peanut butter	160 mL
1¾ cups	milk, at room temperature	435 mL
2	whole eggs, at room temperature	2
2	egg yolks, at room temperature	2
⅓ cup	sugar	80 mL
2 tsp	vanilla extract	10 mL
6 cups	cubed egg bread	1.5 L
⅔ cup	raspberry or other fruit jam	160 mL
	turbinado sugar, for sprinkling	

Preheat the oven to 350°F (180°C).

Melt the butter and brush a 9-inch (23 cm) square pan with half of it. Add the peanut butter to the remaining melted butter and heat over low heat until fluid. Remove the pot from the heat and whisk in the milk, then the eggs, egg yolks, sugar, and vanilla. Toss this mixture with the diced bread and let it sit for 10 minutes. Spoon the mixture into the prepared pan and dollop jam over the bread, pressing it in slightly to incorporate it just a touch. Sprinkle the bread with turbinado sugar. Place the pan inside a larger baking dish and fill it with an inch (2.5 cm) of hot tap water. Bake for about 50 minutes, until the pudding is golden on top and set. Let the pudding sit for at least 30 minutes before serving.

This can be served warm or chilled.

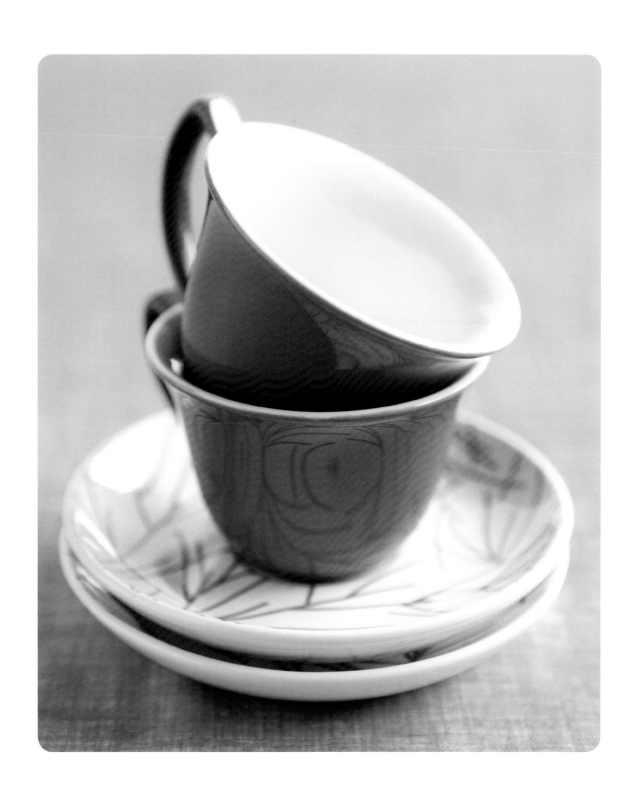

CREAMY TIRAMISU PUDDING *Serves 6*

The original tiramisu is truly spectacular, but is definitely a labor of love. This homemade pudding has all the key elements of tiramisu but is simpler and more casual.

FRESH TAKE

- I made this pudding in tribute to my good friends Mike and Tina. Tiramisu is their absolute favorite, so I first made this when they came over for a Tuesday-night supper.

- This recipe follows a standard pudding or pastry cream technique. When I make a pastry cream, I usually fold in a little whipped cream at the end, after the pastry cream has cooled. In this version, I take advantage of tiramisu's best ingredient, mascarpone, to really get that creaminess I crave.

- I like to layer this pudding in glasses so you can really appreciate the coffee layer on top of the rich chocolate layer.

4 cups	2% milk, divided	1 L
2 tsp	instant coffee	10 mL
4	large egg yolks	4
¼ cup	cornstarch	60 mL
½ cup	sugar	125 mL
1 tsp	vanilla extract	5 mL
2 oz	bittersweet chocolate, chopped	60 g
1 cup	mascarpone cheese	250 mL
	ground cinnamon and cocoa powder, for garnish	

Heat 3 cups (750 mL) of the milk and the instant coffee until just below a simmer. In a bowl, whisk the remaining 1 cup (250 mL) milk, egg yolks, and cornstarch. When the milk is heated, whisk the sugar into the eggs. Slowly whisk the hot milk into the egg mixture, stirring constantly. Return the milk mixture to the pot and whisk over medium heat until thick and glossy, about 5 minutes. Remove the pot from the heat, stir in the vanilla, strain through a sieve, and pour half the mixture over the chopped chocolate, stirring until the chocolate is melted. Place plastic wrap on the surface of both puddings and chill completely.

Stir the mascarpone cheese to soften it then whisk it into the coffee pudding. To assemble, spoon chocolate pudding into 6 serving glasses. Spoon coffee pudding over the chocolate pudding and garnish with a sprinkle of cinnamon and a dusting of cocoa powder.

MINI LEMON MERINGUE CHEESECAKES

Makes about 4 dozen mini cheesecakes

Lemon meringue pie meets cheesecake, and in little bites that make you believe they're low in calories. What a crowd pleaser!

FRESH TAKE

· Baking these cheesecakes in paper liners, like cupcakes, is brilliant. The cheesecakes are easy to remove from the pan, pretty to present on a tiered plate, and tidy to pick up and eat.

· When dealing with such small proportions, a little lemon goes a long way for big flavor. The 1 Tbsp (15 mL) of zest provides the pleasant and lingering lemon taste, while the 2 Tbsp (30 mL) of juice provides just the right tartness.

· Testing the doneness of mini cheesecakes is the same as checking a full-sized version, though they take a fraction of the time to cook. A set surface with a little jiggle in the middle is the surest sign of a properly cooked cheesecake.

Crust

1½ cups	graham cracker crumbs	375 mL
¼ cup	unsalted butter, melted	60 mL
1½ Tbsp	sugar	22.5 mL

Cheesecake

2	8 oz (225 g) pkgs cream cheese, at room temperature	2
⅔ cup	sugar	160 mL
2 Tbsp	cornstarch	30 mL
1 Tbsp	finely grated lemon zest	15 mL
2 Tbsp	lemon juice	30 mL
2 tsp	vanilla extract	10 mL
2	large eggs, at room temperature	2

Meringue

2	large egg whites	2
¼ tsp	lemon juice	1 mL
3 Tbsp	sugar	45 mL
1½ tsp	cornstarch	7.5 mL

Preheat the oven to 350°F (180°C). Line four 12-cup mini muffin tins (48 cups) with paper liners.

For the crust, combine all the ingredients until they're evenly blended and crumbly. Press the crumbs into the bottom of the mini muffin cups. Bake for 8 minutes, then cool.

For the cheesecake, reduce the oven temperature to 325°F (160°C). Beat the cream cheese until smooth and fluffy, then gradually add the sugar while still beating, scraping the sides of the bowl often. Beat in the cornstarch, lemon zest, lemon juice, and vanilla. Add the eggs one at a time, scraping well after each addition. Spoon or pipe cheesecake filling into the cooled mini muffin tins and bake for about 18 minutes, until the cheesecake still moves a little when the pan is shaken gently. Let the cheesecakes cool to room temperature, then chill for at least 2 hours.

Continued . . .

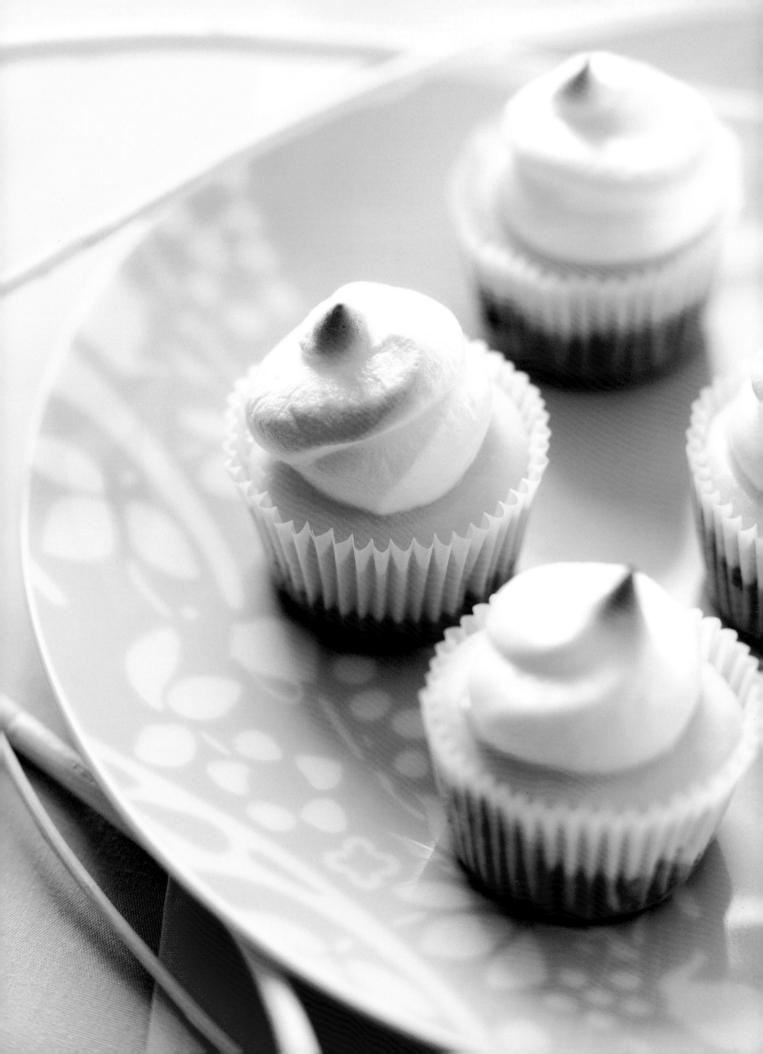

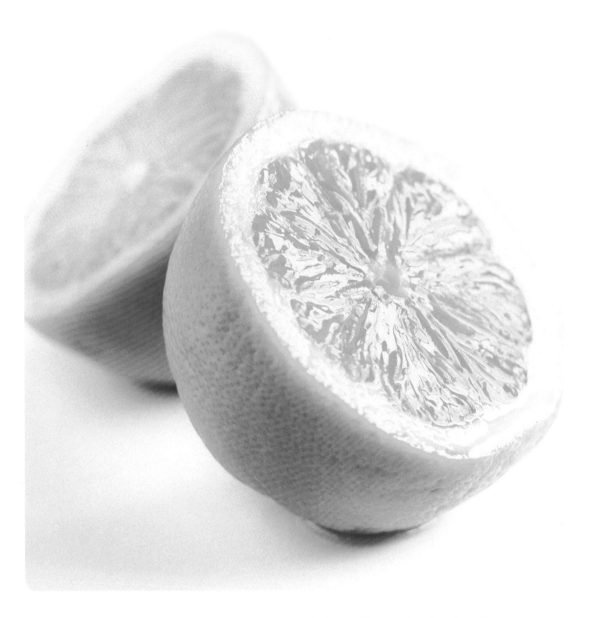

Mini Lemon Meringue Cheesecakes (continued)

For the meringue, preheat the oven to 375°F (190°C).
With an electric mixer, whip the egg whites with the lemon juice until foamy. While whipping, gradually pour in the sugar and whip on one speed less than highest until the whites hold a stiff peak (the meringue stands upright when the whisk is lifted). Whisk in the cornstarch. Fill a piping bag fitted with a large star or plain tip and pipe on top of each cheesecake. Bake for about 6 minutes, just until the meringue browns lightly. Allow the cheesecakes to chill for at least an hour and up to a day before serving.

VERY VANILLA CUPCAKES *Makes 3 dozen mini cupcakes*

Good from-scratch cupcakes are fun to make, but even more fun is decorating them after they've been iced.

FRESH TAKE

· These are a lovely, very white cupcake. They'll be done baking and spring back when touched before they show even a hint of browning. Let your fingers, not your eyes, be your guide.

· I like to use vanilla bean paste (or, alternatively, seeds from a vanilla bean) in this recipe because I appreciate the visual impact of the little seeds scattered throughout the cake and icing. If you can't find vanilla bean paste, use the same measure of pure vanilla extract.

· You can decorate the cupcakes as you choose, or set out a buffet of colored decorations for people to decorate their own—a perfect activity for a kid's birthday party or theme event.

½ cup	cake flour	125 mL
6 Tbsp	all-purpose flour	90 mL
1 tsp	baking powder	5 mL
pinch	fine sea salt	pinch
3 Tbsp	2% milk	45 mL
2 Tbsp	vegetable oil	30 mL
1 tsp	vanilla bean paste, OR scraped seeds from ½ vanilla bean (other ½ for the icing)	5 mL
4	large eggs, separated	4
12 Tbsp	sugar, divided	180 mL

Easy Icing

4 oz	cream cheese, at room temperature	125 g
½ cup	unsalted butter, at room temperature	125 mL
3 cups	icing sugar, sifted	750 mL
1 tsp	vanilla bean paste	5 mL
1–2 Tbsp	milk	15–30 mL

Preheat the oven to 350°F (180°C). Line three 12-cup mini muffin tins (36 cups) with paper liners.

Sift together the flours, baking powder, and salt and set them aside. Whisk together the milk, oil, and vanilla bean paste or seeds and set aside.

Whip the egg whites with 6 Tbsp (90 mL) of the sugar until they hold a soft peak when the beaters are lifted. In a separate bowl, whip the egg yolks with the remaining 6 Tbsp (90 mL) of sugar until they've doubled in volume and have a pale, buttery color. Fold the whipped whites into the yolk mixture then fold in the flour in 2 equal additions. Stir a spoonful of batter into the milk mixture then add this all back to the batter, folding quickly to incorporate. Pipe or spoon the batter into the prepared muffin cups, three-quarters full. Bake for 13 to 15 minutes, until the cupcake springs back when touched. Let cool.

For the icing, use electric beaters to beat the cream cheese and butter until fluffy and smooth. On low speed, add the icing sugar, 1 cup (250 mL) at a time, until blended. Beat in the vanilla bean paste or seeds and add the milk, 1 Tbsp (15 mL) at a time, until the desired consistency is achieved. Ice the cupcakes as desired.

WALNUT TORTE *Makes one 9-inch (23 cm) torte • Serves 12*

This Viennese-style torte is right up my alley. I'm a complete sucker for the elegant, classic tortes of days gone by.

FRESH TAKE

- This style of cake is called a genoise sponge. Whipping the whole eggs with the sugar gives the cake its airy structure, so give the eggs lots of time to whip. Unlike whipping straight egg whites, you can't overwhip whole eggs. The longer you whip, the finer the bubbles in the batter, and the more delicate and tender the cake.

- Pulsing the walnuts with flour for the cake batter protects the batter from the nut oils, keeping the nuts suspended in the cake, not sinking to the bottom.

- The custard icing for this torte tastes like a pastry cream, but sets up like a buttercream. The apricot jam layer in the cake is a Viennese touch, making the torte undeniably elegant.

Cake

1 cup	walnut pieces	250 mL
1 cup	all-purpose flour, divided	250 mL
½ tsp	salt	2 mL
7	large eggs, at room temperature	7
¾ cup	sugar	185 mL
1 tsp	vanilla extract	5 mL

Icing

1 cup	2% milk	250 mL
3 Tbsp	custard powder	45 mL
¼ cup	honey	60 mL
2 Tbsp	brandy	30 mL
1 tsp	vanilla extract	5 mL
2 cups	walnut pieces (more for garnish)	500 mL
1 cup	icing sugar, sifted	250 mL
1½ cups	unsalted butter, at room temperature	375 mL
½ cup	apricot jam	125 mL
	chopped walnuts and walnut halves, for garnish	

Preheat the oven to 350°F (180°C). Grease a 9-inch (23 cm) springform pan, dust it with sugar tapping out any excess, and line the bottom with parchment paper.

For the cake, pulse the nuts with ½ cup (125 mL) flour until fine. Sift the remaining ½ cup (125 mL) flour with the salt and stir in the nut mixture. Set aside.

Whip the eggs, sugar, and vanilla in a mixer, or with electric beaters, until the mixture holds a ribbon when the beaters are lifted, about 6 minutes. In 2 equal additions, fold in the walnut mixture, then pour it into the prepared pan. Bake for 35 to 40 minutes, or until a tester inserted in the center of the cake comes out clean. Cool the cake in the pan on a rack for 15 minutes, then remove it from the pan to cool completely.

For the icing, whisk the milk and custard powder in a small saucepot and bring it up to a simmer, whisking constantly until thick, about 4 minutes. Whisk in the honey quickly and remove the pot from the heat. Strain through a sieve into a bowl, then sit this bowl inside another bowl with ice water to halt the cooking process. Stir in the brandy and vanilla and cool to room temperature, stirring occasionally.

While the custard is cooling, pulse the walnut pieces and icing sugar in a food processor then set the mix aside.

Place the custard in a mixer fitted with the paddle attachment and beat until smooth. Add the butter a little at a time, scraping down the sides of the bowl often. Once the butter has been incorporated, reduce the speed and add the nut mixture, mixing until blended.

To assemble the cake, cut the walnut torte in half, placing one half on a serving plate. Spread apricot jam overtop, then spread about ¾ cup (185 mL) of the walnut icing on top. Put the top half in place and ice the top and sides, covering the cake completely. Gently press the chopped walnuts into the sides of the cake. Garnish the top of the cake with walnut halves and chill.

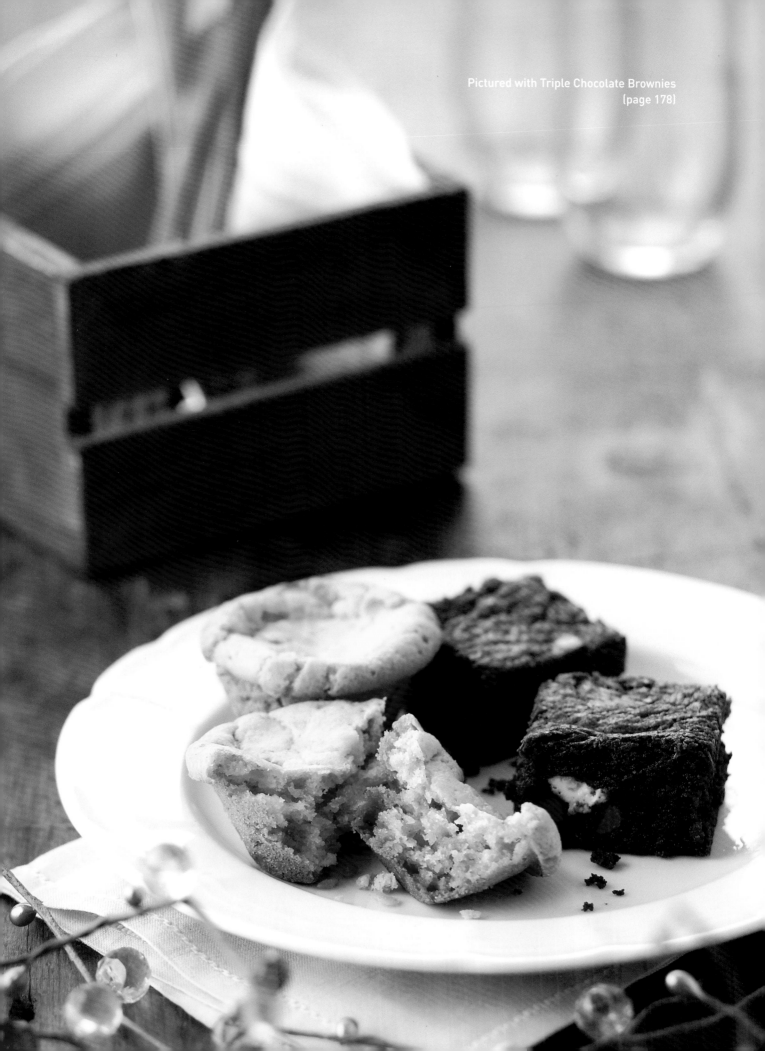

Pictured with Triple Chocolate Brownies
(page 178)

BUTTERSCOTCH WHITE CHOCOLATE BROWNIE BITES

Makes one 9- × 13-inch (23 × 33 cm) pan or 3 dozen mini muffin-sized bites

These are sweet, **sweet,** *SWEET! Melting toffee bits into buttery white-chocolate brownies makes for a great sugar rush.*

FRESH TAKE

- One of the basic rules of dark chocolate brownies is to avoid working in too much air in order to make them fudgy and not cake-like, which is done by mixing carefully by hand and by not using baking powder. White chocolate brownies, however, break this rule. They do need that lift of whipped eggs and baking powder to keep them from being too heavy.

- A great option in place of the Skor bits? Peanut butter chips!

- White chocolate is made up mostly of cocoa butter, and melts at a lower temperature than milk or dark chocolate. Don't worry if the white chocolate and butter mixture looks a little curdled once melted—it will incorporate into the brownies just fine.

⅓ cup	unsalted butter, cut into pieces	80 mL
6 oz	white chocolate, chopped	175 g
2	eggs, at room temperature	2
½ cup	packed light brown sugar	125 mL
⅓ cup	sugar	80 mL
1 tsp	vanilla extract	5 mL
1 cup + 2 Tbsp	all-purpose flour	250 mL + 30 mL
½ tsp	baking powder	2 mL
¼ tsp	salt	1 mL
¾ cup	Skor toffee bits	185 mL

Preheat the oven to 350°F (180°C). Grease a 9- × 13-inch (23 × 33 cm) pan and line it with parchment paper so that it hangs over the sides of the pan, or fill three 12-cup mini muffin tins with liners.

Over a pot of barely simmering water melt the butter for 1 minute, then add the chocolate and stir gently until melted. Remove the chocolate from the heat to cool for 5 minutes.

Whip the eggs with the sugars using electric beaters until thick and frothy. By hand, stir in the melted chocolate. In a separate bowl, stir together the flour, baking powder, and salt, then gently stir it into the chocolate mixture. Stir in the Skor bits and spoon the batter into the prepared pan or tins. Bake for 18 to 20 minutes, until it's a rich golden color. Cool to room temperature before removing from the pan.

For a fancier treat, dip each square halfway in melted white chocolate and chill to set.

TRIPLE CHOCOLATE BROWNIES

Makes one 8-inch (20 cm) square pan (or 16 brownies)

A good brownie should satisfy the deepest chocolate craving, and this one does the trick for me every time. (Pictured on page 176.)

(Pictured on page 176.)

FRESH TAKE

- I have to confess that I typically don't gravitate toward brownies with walnuts in them, even though they are a usual staple ingredient. The addition of the white and milk chocolate pieces gives the brownie a little texture but still keeps this "chocolate focused."

- Room-temperature eggs are important when working with melted chocolate. A cold egg added to warm melted chocolate would seize up the chocolate, resulting in a batter that would be hard to mix, and in brownies that may crumble after they're baked.

10 oz	bittersweet or semisweet chocolate, chopped	300 g
⅔ cup	unsalted butter	160 mL
¾ cup	sugar	180 mL
1 tsp	vanilla extract	5 mL
3	large eggs, at room temperature	3
½ cup	all-purpose flour	125 mL
½ tsp	salt	2 mL
3 oz	white chocolate chips or chunks	90 g
3 oz	milk chocolate chips or chunks	90 g

Preheat the oven to 325°F (160°C). Grease and line an 8-inch (20 cm) square pan with parchment paper.

In a bowl resting over a pot of barely simmering water (but not touching), melt the chopped chocolate and the butter, stirring gently. Remove from the heat and stir in the sugar and vanilla. Stir in the eggs, one at a time, then stir in the flour and salt. Fold in the white and milk chocolate chips or chunks.

Bake for 35 to 40 minutes, until a tester inserted in the center of the brownies comes out clean. Cool before slicing.

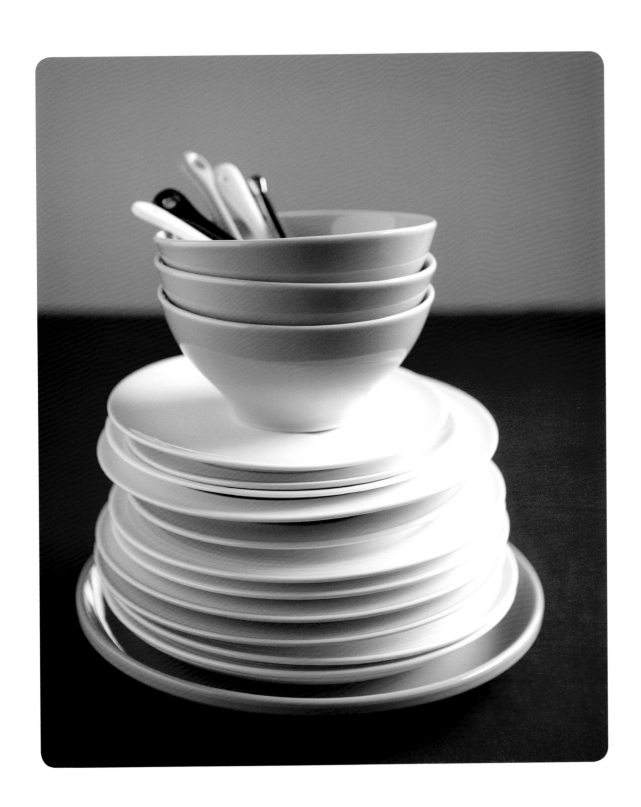

SNACKS FOR ALL SEASONS

There's always a need for snacks, regardless of what time of year it is. A handful of this, a nibble of that—we sometimes eat snacks without even thinking about them.

Well, these snacks will snap you to attention, but that won't stop you from taking that second bite, third bite . . .

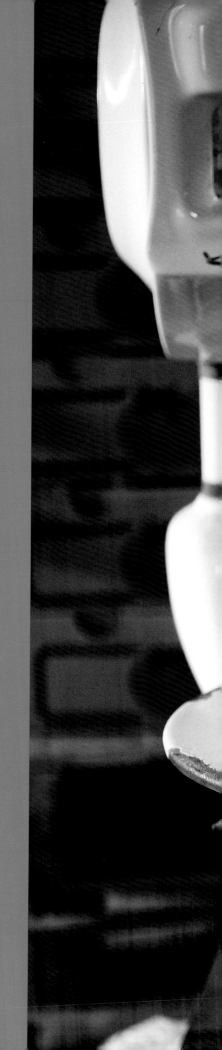

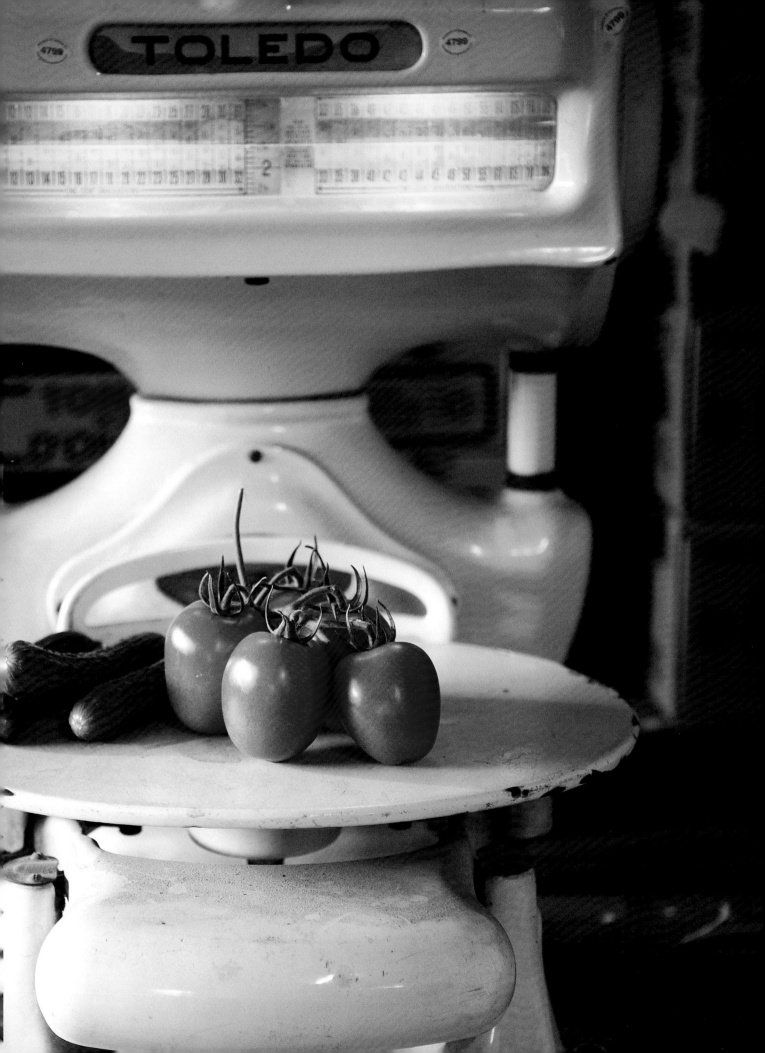

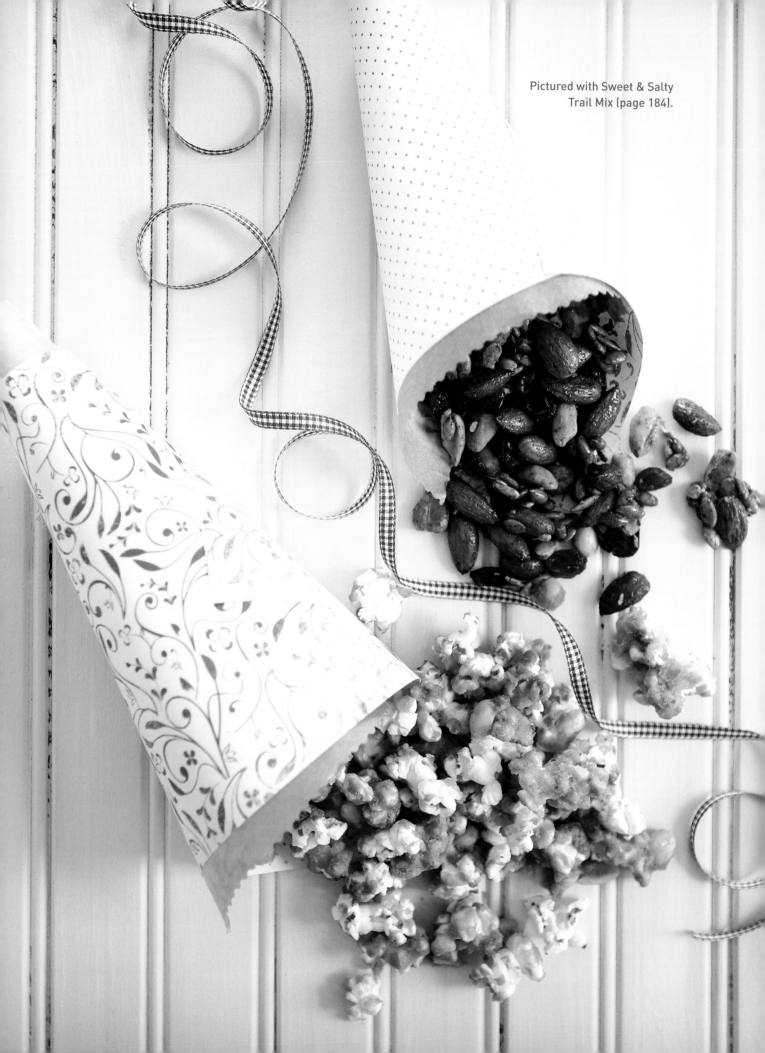

Pictured with Sweet & Salty
Trail Mix (page 184).

CARAMEL PEANUT POPCORN *Makes about 7 cups (1.75 L)*

Salty and sweet is such a hot combination, but be careful. Once you start snacking, you won't be able to stop.

FRESH TAKE

- The maple makes it! Maple syrup has a depth of flavor that makes every biteful satisfying without being cloyingly sweet.

- Any tender nut could be used in place of peanuts, such as pecans or even cashews. If you've purchased unsalted nuts, you may have to add an extra ½ tsp (2 mL) salt to compensate.

- One of my housemates in university introduced me to the magic of salty sweet popcorn. She used to just toss popcorn with salt, cooked sugar, and a little vinegar, and it immediately became my studytime staple (with the occasional soap opera break).

5 cups	popped popcorn kernels	1.25 L
2 cups	salted peanuts	500 mL
1¼ cups	packed light brown sugar	310 mL
¼ cup	unsalted butter	60 mL
¼ cup	pure maple syrup	60 mL
2 tsp	vanilla extract	10 mL
1 tsp	white vinegar	5 mL
½ tsp	salt	2 mL
¼ tsp	baking soda	1 mL

Preheat the oven to 250°F (120°C). Line a baking tray with parchment paper.

Toss the popcorn and peanuts on the tray and keep them warm in the oven while you prepare the caramel.

In a saucepot over medium-low heat, stir the brown sugar, butter, and maple syrup until the butter is melted. Increase the heat to high and boil the sugar mixture until a candy thermometer reads 255°F (124°C) (just past the soft-ball stage), about 4 minutes. While the mixture is boiling, occasionally brush the insides of the pot with a pastry or silicone brush dipped in cool water. Remove the pot from the heat and stir in the vanilla extract, vinegar, salt, and baking soda (the mixture will bubble). Slowly pour the syrup over the popcorn and peanuts, gently stirring to coat the popcorn completely.

Bake until the caramel feels dry, stirring occasionally, about 1 hour 20 minutes. Remove the tray from the oven then use a metal spatula to loosen the mixture from the pan. Cool completely in the pan.

Caramel peanut popcorn will keep for up to 1 week if stored in an airtight container.

SWEET & SALTY TRAIL MIX *Makes about 4 cups (1 L)*

Hhhmmmm . . . I'm sensing a theme here in my snack choices. Like the caramel peanut popcorn (previous page), it's the contrasting mix that makes this the ideal snack. (Pictured on page 182.)

FRESH TAKE

- I sneak pumpkin seeds into things whenever I can. They have a particularly nice nuttiness that's a little more subtle than sunflower seeds. They're a great replacement for nuts in things like muffins or oatmeal cookies, too.

- Because I'm mixing salty and sweet here, I like to mix in spices from both sides of the spectrum. The cinnamon plays against the celery salt and cumin to really balance every bite.

- I always chuckle at the term "trail mix"—I envision myself lost in the woods somewhere, having to rely on my camping skills and a pocketful of trail mix to survive. Thank goodness for the trail mix, because with my camping skills I wouldn't last two hours.

1 cup	whole almonds	250 mL
1 cup	unsalted peanuts	250 mL
½ cup	shelled unsalted pumpkin seeds	125 mL
¼ cup	unsalted sunflower seeds	60 mL
3 Tbsp	pure maple syrup	45 mL
1 tsp	celery salt	5 mL
½ tsp	coarse sea salt	2 mL
½ tsp	ground cumin	2 mL
¼ tsp	ground cinnamon	1 mL
½ cup	raisins	125 mL
½ cup	dried cranberries	125 mL

Preheat the oven to 375°F (190°C). Line a baking tray with parchment paper.

Toss the almonds, peanuts, pumpkin seeds, and sunflower seeds with the maple syrup, celery salt, sea salt, cumin, and cinnamon. Spread everything onto the prepared baking tray and bake, stirring once, for 18 to 20 minutes, until the nuts are toasted. While it's still warm, stir in the raisins and cranberries. Let the trail mix cool.

Store in an airtight container for up to 3 weeks.

SESAME PUMPKIN SEED SNAPS *Makes about 3 dozen snaps*

Sesame comes alive in these sweet little bites, which are great for after-school snacks or to pack in lunches.

FRESH TAKE

· Ever bought those sesame cookies at the corner store or gas station? Sometimes they just hit the spot. They're my inspiration for this homemade version.

· A flexible silicone mini muffin pan works best so you can easily pop out the snaps. If you don't have one, line your metal mini muffin tin with paper liners and spoon the batter into them. You can either store the snaps in the paper cups or just peel away the paper after baking.

1¼ cups	sugar	310 mL
1 cup	unsalted pumpkin seeds	250 mL
¾ cup	sesame seeds, lightly toasted	185 mL
¾ cup	all-purpose flour	185 mL
⅓ cup	vegetable oil	80 mL
¼ cup	pure maple syrup	60 mL
1 Tbsp	finely grated orange zest	15 mL
1½ Tbsp	orange juice	22.5 mL
1½ Tbsp	lemon juice	22.5 mL

Preheat the oven to 350°F (180°C). Grease a silicone mini muffin tray and place it on a metal baking tray.

Blend together the sugar, pumpkin seeds, sesame seeds, and flour. In a separate bowl, whisk the oil, maple syrup, orange zest and juice, and lemon juice to combine then stir the mix into the flour mixture until evenly blended. Spoon a scant teaspoon (5 mL) of batter into the prepared pan and spread it out evenly; wet your fingers with water to press it in. (You may have to do this in batches. You will end up with about 36 snaps.) Bake for 15 to 17 minutes, until the snaps are golden brown and bubbling at the edges. Let them cool completely before popping them out of the muffin tin.

CHEDDAR CRACKERS *Makes 64 crackers*

Homemade crackers are a worthwhile treat, and make a great hostess gift.

FRESH TAKE

· I've tried making crackers a fair bit over the years, often with tough or chewy results. This recipe impresses me with its tenderness and ease in rolling.

· You can switch out the cheddar for another aged cheese like Asiago or Romano—just adjust the water as needed so that it makes a soft, rollable dough.

¾ cup	all-purpose flour	185 mL
¼ cup	cornmeal	60 mL
1 Tbsp	sesame seeds (more for sprinkling)	15 mL
¼ tsp	salt	1 mL
¼ tsp	baking powder	1 mL
¼ cup	unsalted butter, frozen	60 mL
1 cup	coarsely grated old or extra-old cheddar	250 mL
1	egg whisked with 2 Tbsp (30 mL) water, for brushing	1
	coarse salt and sesame seeds, for sprinkling	

In a food processor pulse together the flour, cornmeal, sesame seeds, salt, and baking powder. Use a box grater to grate in the butter and pulse until the mixture is rough and crumbly. Add the cheddar cheese and ¼ cup (60 mL) cold water and pulse until the water is incorporated, adding another 1 Tbsp (15 mL) water if necessary to form a soft dough.

On a lightly floured work surface, knead the dough 3 or 4 times to develop the gluten in the flour slightly and make the dough easier to work with. Form the dough into 2 balls and flatten them into disks and chill for at least an hour.

Preheat the oven to 400°F (200°C). Line a baking tray with parchment paper.

On a lightly floured surface, roll out the first piece of dough into a 12-inch (30 cm) square (about ¹⁄₁₆ inch/2 mm thick) and cut it into 2-inch (5 cm) squares. Place the squares on the prepared baking tray. Repeat with the second piece of dough.

Brush the squares lightly with egg wash and prick them all over with a fork. Sprinkle them with salt and sesame seeds and bake until lightly browned, about 13 minutes. Cool before transferring them to a plate.

These crackers can be stored for up to 5 days in an airtight container.

RED LENTIL DAL *Makes about 2½ cups (625 mL)*

This fragrant stew is an Indian staple. I like to serve it warm with warm naan, or it can be a great alternative to hummus with veggies.

2 Tbsp	vegetable oil or ghee	30 mL
2 cups	diced onion	500 mL
3 cloves	garlic, minced	3 cloves
1 cup	red lentils, rinsed	250 mL
1 tsp	ground cumin	5 mL
½ tsp	turmeric powder	2 mL
	salt & pepper	
¼ cup	chopped cilantro	60 mL

In a medium saucepot, heat the oil or ghee over medium heat. Add the onion and sauté for 4 minutes, until translucent. Add the garlic and sauté for 1 minute more. Add the lentils, 3 cups (750 mL) water, cumin, and turmeric and bring everything up to a simmer, stirring occasionally. Simmer for about 15 minutes, until the lentils are tender.

Transfer half the mixture to a food processor or blender and purée until smooth. Stir the puréed mixture back into the pot, season to taste, and serve warm or at room temperature, topped with fresh cilantro.

TONNATO DIP *Makes about 1 cup (250 mL)*

Vitello tonnato is one of my favorite Italian dishes. It's the creamy sauce that tops chilled, poached veal and it's salty and satisfying. As a dip, it's just as tasty.

FRESH TAKE

- Quality tuna counts here, since it's the key ingredient. I buy good Italian tuna packed in oil. Once it's puréed with the other ingredients, it smoothes out to a perfect creamy consistency.

- When I need to build a make-your-own sandwich buffet, I like to include dips such as this as an alternative to mayonnaise and mustard. A spoonful of this spread on a ciabatta bun with cold roasted pork or chicken and a few leaves of radicchio is a thing of beauty.

- If I need a packed lunch or eat on the go, I'm inclined to opt for this and a side container of veggies over a tuna sandwich. (But not in my car—too messy.)

2	3 oz (80 g) cans tuna in oil	2
3 Tbsp	minced sweet onion	45 mL
2 Tbsp	lemon juice	30 mL
4 Tbsp	capers, divided	60 mL
1 Tbsp	juice from caper jar	15 mL
2 tsp	anchovy paste	10 mL
¼ cup	olive oil	60 mL
	salt & pepper	

In a food processor, purée the tuna with the onion, lemon juice, 2 Tbsp (30 mL) of the capers, caper juice, and anchovy paste until smooth. Pour in the olive oil in a thin stream while the blender is running. Season to taste and chill until ready to serve.

LEMON HUMMUS with PITA *Makes about 2 cups (500 ml)*

There's no need to buy hummus when it's so easy to make at home.

FRESH TAKE
- Tahini paste is simply ground sesame seeds. It can be found at most grocery stores these days (just like premade hummus!). Try mixing tahini with lemon juice, water, and a little olive oil for a creamy salad dressing, or with a little lemon juice and honey to baste onto grilled chicken.

- Serve a group of dips with cold roasted chicken, bread, and other condiments for an easy and not-too-heavy buffet. This is great after a day of skiing in winter or a day at the beach in summer! It can all be prepared ahead of time, so it's ready for you when you get home.

1	19 oz (540 mL) can chickpeas, drained and rinsed	1
1 clove	garlic, minced	1 clove
3 Tbsp	tahini sesame paste	45 mL
2 Tbsp	lemon juice	30 mL
2 Tbsp	olive oil	30 mL
3 Tbsp	chopped flat-leaf parsley, plus extra for garnish	45 mL
	salt & pepper	
6	small pita, cut into thirds	6
	shredded cooked chicken	

Purée the chickpeas with the garlic, tahini, lemon juice, and olive oil until smooth, adding cold water as needed until you have your desired consistency. Stir in the chopped parsley, season, and chill until ready to serve.

To serve, cut open a pita and spoon in some shredded chicken. Add a spoonful of hummus and sprinkle with parsley.

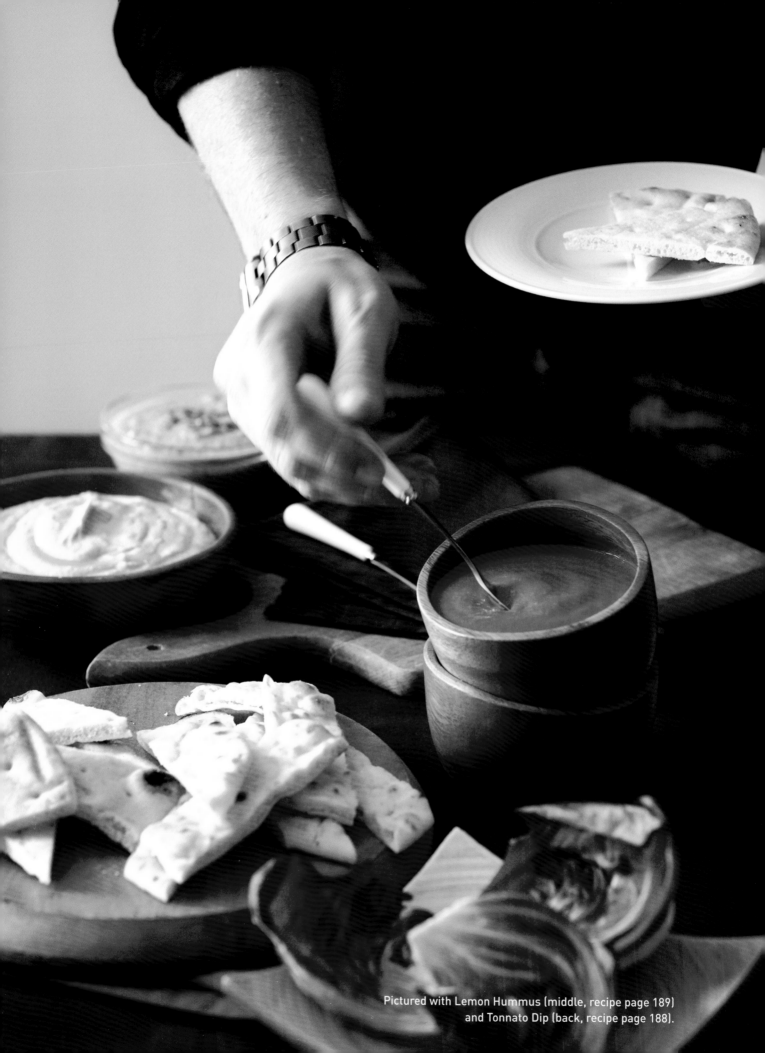

Pictured with Lemon Hummus (middle, recipe page 189)
and Tonnato Dip (back, recipe page 188).

EASY PEPPER DIP *Makes about 1 cup (250 ml)*

What a way to end the book—with the easiest recipe ever!

- Feel free to roast your own peppers and then purée them. You can grill two bell peppers on high then place them in a covered bowl to cool. Peel off the skin and remove the seeds, then away you go!

- The amount of oil you add to the recipe is up to you, according to your taste. The more oil you drizzle in, the creamier the consistency.

- This is a colorful appetizer dip, but if you add a little water it also makes a great sauce served warm or at room temperature over cooked green beans or asparagus.

1	13 fl oz (375 mL) jar roasted bell peppers, drained	1
1 clove	garlic, minced	1 clove
	olive oil	
	salt & pepper	

Purée the roasted peppers with the garlic until smooth. Drizzle in just a touch of olive oil while puréeing, until you have your desired consistency (thicker than a sauce), then season to taste and chill until ready to serve.

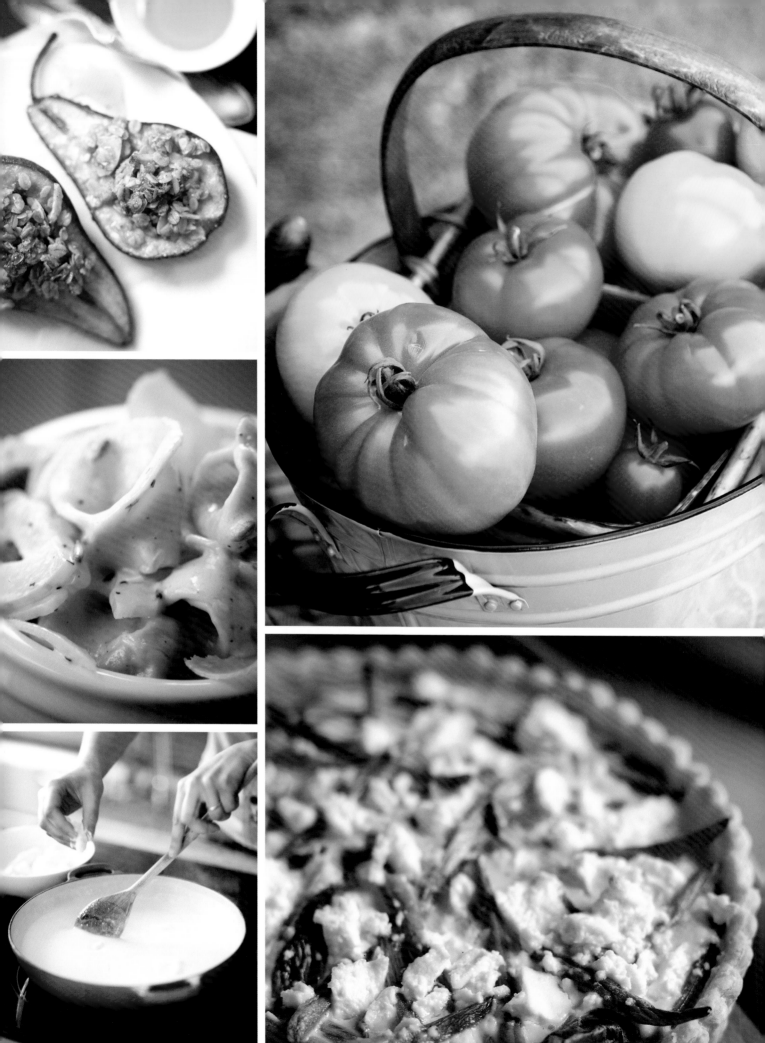

INDEX

WELCOME BACK

HELP YOURSELF! PLEASE BE HON[EST]

PLEASE USE THE BAGS PROVID[ED]

THANK YOU VERY MUCH !!!!

THE MUILE BOOM

2.50

2.50